Improving the quality and use of birth, death and cause-of-death information:
guidance for a standards-based review of country practices

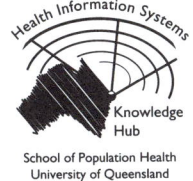
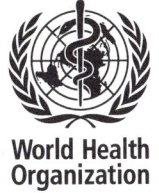

WHO Library Cataloguing-in-Publication Data

Improving the quality and use of birth, death and cause-of-death information: guidance for a standards-based review of country practices

1.Civil registration. 2.Vital statistics. 3.Birth rate. 4.Mortality. 5.Cause of death. 6.Pregnancy rate. 7.Data collection – standards. 8.National health programmes – standards. I.World Health Organization.

ISBN 978 92 4 154797 0   (NLM classification: WA 900)

© World Health Organization 2010

All rights reserved. Publications of the World Health Organization can be obtained from WHO Press, World Health Organization, 20 Avenue Appia, 1211 Geneva 27, Switzerland (tel.: +41 22 791 3264; fax: +41 22 791 4857; e-mail: bookorders@who.int). Requests for permission to reproduce or translate WHO publications – whether for sale or for noncommercial distribution – should be addressed to WHO Press, at the above address (fax: +41 22 791 4806; e-mail: permissions@who.int).

The designations employed and the presentation of the material in this publication do not imply the expression of any opinion whatsoever on the part of the World Health Organization concerning the legal status of any country, territory, city or area or of its authorities, or concerning the delimitation of its frontiers or boundaries. Dotted lines on maps represent approximate border lines for which there may not yet be full agreement.

The mention of specific companies or of certain manufacturers' products does not imply that they are endorsed or recommended by the World Health Organization in preference to others of a similar nature that are not mentioned. Errors and omissions excepted, the names of proprietary products are distinguished by initial capital letters.

All reasonable precautions have been taken by the World Health Organization to verify the information contained in this publication. However, the published material is being distributed without warranty of any kind, either expressed or implied. The responsibility for the interpretation and use of the material lies with the reader. In no event shall the World Health Organization be liable for damages arising from its use.

Printed in Malta by Progress Press Co. Ltd.

Editing and production by Cadman Editing Services, Canberra

Designed by Robert Redding

Acknowledgements

This document is the result of collaboration by a broad range of public health experts. Lene Mikkelsen and Alan Lopez – from the School of Population Health, University of Queensland, Australia – co-wrote the original text. Valuable inputs to early drafts were provided by Vicki Bennett (School of Population Health, University of Queensland, Australia), Debbie Bradshaw (Medical Research Council, Cape Town, South Africa), John Cleland (London School of Hygiene and Tropical Medicine, London, United Kingdom), Francesca Grum (United Nations Statistics Division, New York, United States), Rafael Lozano (Institute for Health Metrics and Evaluation at the University of Washington, United States); Prasantha Mahapatra (Institute of Health Systems, Hyderabad, Andhra Pradesh, India), Cleone Rooney (Office of National Statistics, London, United Kingdom), Kenji Shibuya (University of Tokyo, Tokyo, Japan), Sue Walker (School of Public Health, Queensland University of Technology, Australia) and Eduardo Zacca (Ministry of Health, Havana, Cuba).

Particular thanks are due to the following country partners who tested the approach and provided valuable feedback: Estuardo Albán (Instituto Nacional de Estadistica y Censos, Ecuador), Lourdes J Hufana (National Statistical Office, Manila), Charity Tan (Department of Health, the Philippines) and Rasika Rampatige (Ministry of Health, Sri Lanka).

Important contributions were also provided by the following World Health Organization (WHO) staff: Mohamed Ali (WHO Eastern Mediterranean Region, Cairo, Egypt), Mark Amexo (Health Metrics Network, WHO, Geneva, Switzerland), Jun Gao (WHO Western Pacific Region, Manila, Philippines), Alejandro Giusti (WHO Region of the Americas, Santiago, Chile), Fiona Gore (WHO, Geneva, Switzerland), Mie Inoue (WHO, Geneva, Switzerland), Robert Jakob (WHO, Geneva, Switzerland), Enrique Loyola (WHO European Region, Copenhagen, Denmark), Doris MaFat (WHO, Geneva, Switzerland), Fatima Marinho (WHO/Pan American Health Organization, Washington DC, United States), Lucille Nievera (WHO Country Office, Manila, the Philippines), Sunil Senanayake (WHO South-East Asia Region, Delhi, India) and William Soumbey-Alley (WHO African Region, Brazzaville, Congo).

Carla AbouZahr (WHO, Geneva, Switzerland) oversaw the development of the tool, with administrative assistance from Sue Piccolo and Petra Schuster. Financial support was provided by the Government of Japan, the Health Metrics Network of the WHO and the Health Information Systems Hub at the School of Population Health at the University of Queensland.

Abbreviations and acronyms

ACME	Automated Classification of Medical Entities
AIDS	acquired immunodeficiency syndrome
DHS	Demographic and Health Surveys
DOA	dead on arrival
HIV	human immunodeficiency virus
HMN	Health Metrics Network
ICD-10	International statistical classification of diseases and related health problems, 10th revision
MICS	Multiple Indicators Cluster Survey
MDG	Millennium Development Goal (United Nations)
MoVE	monitoring of vital events
NGO	nongovernmental organization
PAHO	Pan American Health Organization
PAPCHILD	Pan Arab Project for Child Development
SAVVY	sample vital registration with verbal autopsy
UN	United Nations
UNICEF	United Nations Children's Fund
UNFPA	United Nations Population Fund
UNSD	United Nations Statistics Division
WHO	World Health Organization

Contents

Acknowledgements iii
Abbreviations and acronyms iv
Executive summary ix

1 Introduction 1
    1.1 What are civil registration and vital statistics systems? 1
    1.2 What is the WHO guidance tool? 2
    1.3 Benefits of using the guidance tool 3
    1.4 Scope 3
    1.5 Audience 4
    1.6 Benefits of, and responsibilities for, civil registration 4
        1.6.1 Individuals 4
        1.6.2 Countries 5
        1.6.3 Summary of uses and benefits 7
    1.7 Global status of civil registration and vital statistics systems 7

2 Process for reviewing civil registration and vital statistics systems 9
    2.1 Step 1 – Form a review committee and raise awareness 10
        2.1.1 Phase 1: Identify a lead agency 10
        2.1.2 Form a review committee 10
        2.1.3 Make a case to government 11
    2.2 Step 2 – Undertake a rapid assessment 11
    2.3 Step 3 – Launch the review 12
        2.3.1 Launch meeting 12
        2.3.2 Subgroups 12
    2.4 Step 4 – Conduct an initial committee meeting 13
    2.5 Step 5 – Conduct work sessions with subgroups 13
    2.6 Phase 2: Step 6 – Conduct a results meeting 14
    2.7 Step 7 – Conduct a review committee meeting to draft a strategic plan 14
    2.8 Step 8 – Conduct a final stakeholder meeting 15
    2.9 Phase 3: Implementation 15
        2.9.1 Towards sustainable civil registration and vital statistics systems 15
        2.9.2 Monitoring progress 15

3	The WHO assessment framework	17
	3.1 Development and structure	17
	3.2 Overview of components and subcomponents of the WHO assessment framework	17
	3.3 Component A – Legal basis and resources for civil registration	18
	3.4 Component B – Registration practices, coverage and completeness	26
	3.5 Component C – Death certification and cause of death	39
	3.6 Component D – ICD mortality coding practices	48
	3.7 Component E – Data access, use and quality checks	53
Annex A	**Strategic planning for strengthening the vital statistics system**	**65**
Annex B	**Template for launch meeting agenda**	**66**
Annex C	**Suggested indicators for monitoring progress in national civil registration and vital statistics systems**	**67**
Annex D	**Leading causes of deaths by age group and income group for both sexes**	**68**
Glossary		73
References		77

Tables

Table 2.1	Scores, ratings and actions required for rapid assessment	12
Table 3.1	Inputs, processes and outputs	17
Table C1	Suggested indicators	67
Table D1	All ages	68
Table D2	Ages 0–9 years	69
Table D3	Ages 10–19 years	70
Table D4	Ages 20–59 years	71
Table D5	Age 60+ years	72

Figures

Figure 1.1	Infant mortality rate by canton, Costa Rica, 2000	6
Figure 1.2	Quality of globally available information on causes of death	8
Figure 3.1	Schematic representation of civil registration and vital statistics systems	20
Figure 3.2	Death registration and certification process in Mexico	27
Figure 3.3	Birth registration process in Mexico	28

Figure A1   Process for preparing a plan to strengthen the vital statistics system 65

Boxes

Box 1.1   Summary of uses of civil registration and vital statistics data 7

Box 2.1   Roadmap of actions and outcomes of the review 9

Box 2.2   Example of distribution of assessment tasks among subgroups 13

Box 3.1   WHO assessment framework 18

Box 3.2   Recommended list of high-priority characteristics to include in birth and death registration information 33

Box 3.3   Access to civil registration and completeness of vital registration 34

Box 3.4   International form of medical certificate of cause of death 40

Box 3.5   Special enquiry systems 42

Box 3.6   Verbal autopsy 45

Box 3.7   Summarized training curriculum for coders 51

Box 3.8   Child mortality in Thailand 54

Box 3.9   Standard plausibility and consistency checks 58

Box 3.10   Percent of deaths expected from three broad cause-of-death groups (I–III) as a function of increases in life expectancy 60

Box 3.11   Typical age pattern of broad cause-of-death groups (I–III) 61

Subcomponents

Subcomponent A1: National legal framework for civil registration and vital statistics systems 21

Subcomponent A2: Registration infrastructure and resources 24

Subcomponent B1: Organization and functioning of civil registration and vital statistics systems 29

Subcomponent B2: Review of forms used for birth and death registration 32

Subcomponent B3: Coverage and completeness of registration 35

Subcomponent B4: Data storage and transmission 38

Subcomponent C1: ICD-compliant practices for death certification 42

Subcomponent C2: Hospital death certification 44

Subcomponent C3: Deaths occurring outside hospital 45

Subcomponent C4: Practices affecting the quality of cause-of-death data 46

Subcomponent D1: Mortality coding practices 49

Subcomponent D2: Mortality coder qualification and training 50

Subcomponent D3: Quality of mortality coding 52

Improving the quality and use of birth, death and cause-of-death information

Subcomponent E1: Data quality and plausibility checks 57

Subcomponent E1 (A): Levels of fertility and mortality.. 57

Subcomponent E1 (B): Cause of death 59

Subcomponent E2: Data tabulation 62

Subcomponent E3: Data access and dissemination 63

Executive summary

Civil registration systems are used to record vital events – including births, deaths, and marriages – and have the potential to serve as the main source of national vital statistics. However, in many developing countries, civil registration and vital statistics systems are weak or nonexistent; as a result, key demographic, fertility and mortality statistics are not available on a continuous basis and do not cover large segments of the population. A first step in addressing such weaknesses is to undertake a review of current status with a view to identifying areas requiring improvement and prioritizing actions.

This package of materials – referred to as the *World Health Organization (WHO) guidance tool* – provides comprehensive guidance on how to systematically evaluate the quality and functioning of civil registration and vital statistics systems. The package consists of two components: a *detailed assessment tool*, plus a *rapid assessment tool* available as text or as a spreadsheet, for ease of compilation of data. Both tools have been extensively peer reviewed by technical experts, and field tested in three countries. The aim is to help responsible authorities obtain a clear and comprehensive understanding of the strengths and weaknesses of their civil registration and vital statistics systems, and generate the evidence base for corrective action.

The detailed assessment tool reviews the main aspects of the civil registration and vital statistics systems. These include the legal and regulatory framework; registration, certification and coding practices; and the compilation, tabulation and use of the resulting data. The tool comprises both a *roadmap*, which outlines the main steps in conducting the review, starting with the formation of a review committee of key stakeholders, and an *assessment framework*, which serves as a template for the detailed review. The focus throughout is on births, deaths and causes of death, because these are the fundamental events that countries need to know about in order to guide public health programmes, monitor population dynamics and measure key health indicators.

The approach described in this guidance tool is largely directed to those countries where civil registration is established but is subject to inadequacies in terms of coverage, quality or both. Countries where civil registration is not established may find the approach useful, even though not all sections of the assessment framework will be relevant. If the extent of completeness or coverage of the vital statistics data is known, even incomplete information can yield valuable insights on mortality patterns and the main causes of death.

The guidance tool emphasizes the importance of critically evaluating data quality by, for example, carrying out consistency and plausibility checks, and comparing the outputs of the systems with data from other sources on mortality and fertility levels and patterns. Statisticians, health planners and others compiling and analysing vital statistics should be strongly encouraged and helped to develop such critical appraisal skills as an essential component of overall system development.

Countries or local governments using these materials will be better informed about the strengths and weaknesses of their current systems, and will be able to identify the processes or aspects that need to be improved. The outcome should be improved and more useful vital statistics to support health sector reforms and development policies and programmes.

1 Introduction

This chapter sets the context for the package of materials by describing what "civil registration" and "vital statistics systems" are and why they are needed.[1] It also outlines the purpose, scope and audience for the materials. Finally, the chapter summarizes the benefits to be gained from effective civil registration and vital statistics systems, and discusses the status of such systems globally.

1.1 What are civil registration and vital statistics systems?

In most countries, a civil registration system is used to record statistics on "vital events" such as "births", deaths, marriages, divorces and "fetal deaths". This government administrative system creates a permanent record of each event. The records derived from civil registration systems have two main uses:

- They are personal legal documents, required by "citizens" as proof of facts (e.g. age and identity) surrounding events; such documents are used, for example, to:
  - establish family relationships and inheritance rights;
  - provide proof of age and establish rights based on age (e.g. school entry, driving privileges);
  - provide proof of marriage or divorce and the right to marry;
  - provide evidence of death.
- They provide data that form the basis of a country's vital statistics system.

"Vital statistics" are used to derive the fundamental demographic and epidemiological measures that are needed in national planning across multiple sectors, such as education, labour and health. They are also critical for a wide range of government activities (e.g. "population registers" and other administrative registers) and commercial enterprises (e.g. life insurance and marketing of products).

In the health sector, vital statistics form the core of a country's health information system, because they:

- permit understanding of the prevalence and distribution of mortality due to diseases and injury, identification of health inequalities and priorities, monitoring of trends and evaluation of the impact and effectiveness of health programmes;

- provide (when timely and complete) a reliable method for measuring baseline levels and monitoring progress towards global goals, such as the United Nations (UN) Millennium Development Goals (MDGs); they are also important in understanding emerging health challenges due to, for example, noncommunicable diseases, injuries and human immunodeficiency virus/ acquired immunodeficiency syndrome (HIV/AIDS);

- enable tracking of national strategies such as health-sector reform, poverty reduction and development efforts;

- support planning, monitoring and evaluation in decentralized health systems, by providing information on health conditions at a regional and local level.

Civil registration records are the best source of vital statistics because they generate data on a continuous basis and for the whole country, at both national and local levels. However, such systems are often weak or incomplete in developing countries. In countries where the civil registration system lacks complete coverage, or has major deficiencies due to issues of quality and timeliness, it may be necessary, on an interim basis, to use alternative sources to generate vital statistics. Sources for such interim data include "population censuses", "household sample surveys", "demographic surveillance" in sentinel sites and sample registration systems. Although these sources can and do generate measures of vital events, they cannot replace civil registration, which is the only method that collects such information on a continuous basis, and the only source that can provide individuals with a legal document of a vital event.

---

[1] Terms given in quotation marks are explained in the Glossary.

Introduction

Civil registration is defined by the UN as (*1*):

> ... the continuous, permanent, compulsory, and universal recording of the occurrence and characteristics of vital events (live births, deaths, fetal deaths, marriages, and divorces) and other civil status events pertaining to the population as provided by decree, law or regulation, in accordance with the legal requirements in each country.

Development and strengthening of civil registration and vital statistics systems are important for improving the quality of a country's vital statistics, and for using this information to guide policies and programmes. This broader concept has been captured in the UN definition of a vital statistics system as (*1*):

> ... the total process of (a) collecting information by civil registration or enumeration on the frequency or occurrence of specified and defined vital events, as well as relevant characteristics of the events themselves and the person or persons concerned, and (b) compiling, processing, analysing, evaluating, presenting and disseminating these data in statistical form.

It is not possible to establish an effective vital statistics system overnight; it requires political will, stewardship by national authorities, and the trust and collaboration of "civil society", households and the medical professions. Countries with poorly functioning vital statistics systems should therefore view the improvement of those systems as a necessary long-term investment, and as a goal that is achievable if there is sustained political commitment.

A lack of resources has often been cited as the main reason why some low-income countries have poorly performing civil registration systems. Although cost is an important consideration, costs are not an insurmountable barrier to improvement, as shown by a number of relatively low-income countries (e.g. Cuba, Sri Lanka and Uruguay) that have well-functioning civil registration systems to monitor health outcomes and provide reliable population data.

If a country lacks civil registration and vital statistics systems, or has systems that do not produce data of sufficient quality, then costs of social and economic programmes are likely to be higher because of inefficiencies and other wasteful use of resources. Without reliable vital statistics it is difficult for communities, governments, donors and multilateral organizations to effectively undertake and monitor the planning and impact of a whole range of social programmes and health initiatives. Vital statistics are the cornerstone of a country's health information system. If information is lacking on the number of births and deaths, and on sex, age and "cause of death", it is difficult to achieve real progress towards the fundamental goal of any health system, which is to keep people alive and healthy for longer.

1.2 What is the WHO guidance tool?

As part of efforts by the World Health Organization (WHO) Health Metrics Network (HMN) to strengthen national health information, a number of countries have expressed the need for a tool that could be used to review how well their civil registration and vital statistics systems are able to generate useful vital statistics and to identify which part or parts of their national system are deficient and need to be improved. In response, the WHO, working with the University of Queensland in Australia, developed this package of materials – referred to as the *WHO guidance tool* – to provide guidance for a standards-based review of country practices in civil registration and vital statistics.

This document – *the detailed assessment tool* – includes:

■ an introduction to civil registration and vital statistics systems (Chapter 1);

■ a *roadmap*, which outlines the process for reviewing current systems (Chapter 2);

■ an *assessment framework*, which provides a structure for the detailed review (Chapter 3).

Introduction

The accompanying document – *Rapid assessment of national civil registration and vital statistics systems* – provides a *rapid* assessment tool to quickly evaluate the state of the current systems, and make the case for a more detailed assessment. It is available as both text and a spreadsheet, for ease of compilation of data.

The rapid assessment tool was developed because many countries suggested that it would be useful to have some evidence, to make the case to senior management before undertaking a detailed review. Both tools have been extensively peer reviewed by technical experts, and field tested in three countries.

The purpose of reviewing existing systems is not to hold individuals accountable for malfunctions or operational problems in current systems, nor is it to find fault with the performance of people responsible for the operation of the vital statistics and civil registration systems. Rather, the purpose is to provide evidence that countries can use to guide the development of improvement plans. Such evidence can be used, for example, in discussions with donors, governments and development partners, when seeking funding for the strengthening of the national civil registration system.

1.3 Benefits of using the guidance tool

Using the guidance tool will help countries to obtain a clear and comprehensive understanding of current approaches, and provide the evidence base for corrective action. However, the guidance tool alone is not sufficient to enable countries to resolve problems with their civil registration system or the quality of their vital statistics. The principal benefits of using the guidance tool include:

- guidance on best practice, derived from the extensive experience of the WHO and other UN agencies in helping countries to develop health and statistical systems;
- full alignment with the broader HMN Framework for country health information systems (*2*);
- accordance with the multipartner initiative on monitoring of vital events (MoVE – a research initiative launched by HMN partners in 2006 to promote registration systems and alternative ways of gathering information on vital events), incorporating valuable lessons learnt from applied research in many developing countries (*3–7*);
- increased insights into the quality of routinely collected birth, death and cause-of-death statistics;
- a means of obtaining the evidence needed to systematically improve vital statistics and related outputs produced by civil registration and vital statistics systems;
- use of a review process (Chapter 2) that engages and builds consensus among key "stakeholders" around identified priority needs.

1.4 Scope

This WHO guidance tool is only intended for the assessment of key vital statistics derived from civil registration; it is not intended for the assessment of the practices and the quality of data obtained from household surveys, censuses or sample registration. The tool promotes international standards and practices, but does not prescribe what measures and practices countries should adopt to achieve fully functioning civil registration and vital statistics systems. Such measures and practices are best determined locally, because much will depend on the local context, capacity, resources and traditions.

Although the UN considers vital events to comprise "live births", deaths, fetal deaths, marriages and divorces, this guidance tool is concerned only with births, deaths and causes of death (i.e. it does not cover fetal deaths, marriages or divorces). This focus reflects the fact that births, deaths and causes of death are the fundamental events that countries need to know about to guide health programmes, monitor population dynamics and measure key health indicators. Although registration of fetal deaths is clearly important in measuring "perinatal mortality", pregnancy outcome

Improving the quality and use of birth, death and cause-of-death information

Introduction

and quality of prenatal health services, fetal deaths are not included in this tool because few countries are currently able to satisfactorily collect the necessary data. However, in countries where data on fetal deaths and perinatal mortality are routinely collected, additional questions should be included in the review of civil registration and vital statistics systems, to address issues of data quality and reliability.

1.5 Audience

This WHO guidance tool is mainly intended for people responsible for the collection, compilation and use of vital statistics. It will be most useful in countries (or regions within countries) that have a functioning civil registration system but do not get the maximum benefit from their vital statistics systems. For these countries, the case for investing in a functioning vital statistics system is particularly strong, because they already spend considerable amounts of money annually on, for example, salaries of registrars and data coders, and infrastructure, equipment and supplies. Some countries currently have civil registration systems that only produce legal documents, while vital statistics are collected by a parallel system, often under the authority of the ministry of health.

The WHO guidance tool will also be of use to countries with complete registration systems; such countries can use this tool to periodically assess the functioning of their systems and the quality of the data they produce, and to take corrective action where needed.

Countries that have little or no civil registration may find that several sections of the assessment tool cannot be completed because there is too little information to assess. However, they may use those parts of the tool that are relevant, especially in relation to the legal framework. In addition, such countries would benefit from consulting other resources developed by the HMN, such as the MoVE *Monitoring vital events resource kit*, which is available both online and as a CD (*8*). The kit is a compilation of technical documents aimed at facilitating the establishment of demographic surveillance sites. It also provides instructions on how to set up "sample vital registration with verbal autopsy" (SAVVY). A combination of demographic surveillance and sample "vital registration" is not an alternative to a civil registration system, but can provide useful interim measures of fertility and mortality, and can help to build the necessary human resources and skills required to ensure the functioning of a civil registration system.

1.6 Benefits of, and responsibilities for, civil registration

1.6.1 Individuals

Civil registration and vital statistics systems that are of high quality, continuous and well-maintained provide many benefits to individuals and their communities, and to countries, regions and the international community.

For the individual, the main benefits of a civil registration system are the provision of legal status and the official documentation of important life events. For example, birth registration certifies identity and provides legal proof of a person's name, their parents' names and their date and place of birth. As a legal document, a birth certificate serves to define and protect a person's human and civil rights in society. The UN Children's Fund (UNICEF) has extensively documented the impact of non-registration of births (*9*), and has had the right to birth registration enshrined as the first legal recognition of the child in Article 7 of the Convention on the Rights of the Child, which states that:

> ... the child shall be registered immediately after birth and shall have the right from birth to a name, the right to acquire a nationality and, as far as possible, the right to know and be cared for by his or her parents.

Non-registration of a child can have severe negative consequences for a child's fundamental rights to benefits such as identity, inheritance, education, health and social services. Birth registration is thus also part of a broader strategy to ensure that children are less vulnerable to abuse and exploitation, especially if they are separated from their parents. In the absence

Improving the quality and use of birth, death and cause-of-death information

of a functioning birth-registration system, it is difficult for a country to enforce age-related legal rights relating to education, child labour, juvenile justice, early marriage, sexual exploitation, electoral rights and military recruitment. Responding effectively to natural disasters often involves reuniting lost children with their families, demonstrating the importance of a birth certificate.

Countries that are signatories to the Convention on the Rights of the Child are expected to set up systems to register the births of all children without applying discriminatory conditions. Countries should ensure compulsory and timely birth registration for all children within the national territory. In particular, countries should focus attention on children in rural and remote areas, and children from vulnerable and marginalized groups; for example, children born to foreign parents, refugees, immigrants, asylum seekers and internally displaced persons.

UNICEF and some nongovernmental organizations (NGOs) such as Plan International, Save the Children's Fund and World Vision have been particularly active in promoting the individual and human right aspects of civil registration, and have conducted successful campaigns in many countries for universal birth registration. They have also raised awareness of the importance of proof of identity for securing recognition before the law, protecting rights (such as inheritance) and providing access to public services.

1.6.2 Countries

For countries, the major benefit of effective civil registration and vital statistics systems is the role they play in supporting and informing effective planning for social and economic development. If vital statistics are collected from a civil registration system that covers all events (not just a sample), they can provide a reliable basis for small-area information needed to design and implement policies on public health, maternal and child care, family planning, social security, education, housing and economic development. At the local level, accurate population data are essential for planning the needs of the community, and for addressing and monitoring regional inequalities. Figure 1.1 uses the example of Costa Rica to illustrate the use of vital statistics for monitoring differences in "infant mortality" at local levels. Such vital statistics are crucial for developing targeted programmes to improve child survival and for channelling resources to where they are most needed.

Another advantage of effective civil registration and vital statistics systems is that the success of international efforts to control specific diseases is often measured in terms of the reduction in deaths that are due to programme interventions. For example, at least six of the MDGs rely on accurate data on mortality and causes of death in monitoring progress (3). A recent report from the World Bank estimates that a major stumbling block in achieving the MDG health goals in Latin America is that infant and maternal mortality data are incomplete (10). There is increasing evidence that long-term improvements to civil registration systems will provide a more cost-effective way to accurately measure reductions in mortality than relying on separate disease-focused approaches, in which data are collected on specific areas of interest (e.g. HIV/AIDS, malaria, tuberculosis and vaccine-preventable diseases) (7).

Most civil registration systems also collect information on causes of death, although these data are often processed in a country's ministry of health. Statistics based on death records are particularly important for identifying the magnitude and distribution of major diseases, and are essential for the design, implementation, monitoring and assessment of health programmes and policies. For example, statistics on deaths from lung cancer, alcohol-related liver disease and alcohol-related traffic deaths have been important in many countries in establishing legislation to reduce exposure to the harmful effects of tobacco and alcohol. Moreover, because vital statistics are collected on a continuing basis, they are also crucial for detecting and understanding how new health challenges

Introduction

Figure 1.1 Infant mortality rate by cantons, Costa Rica 2000

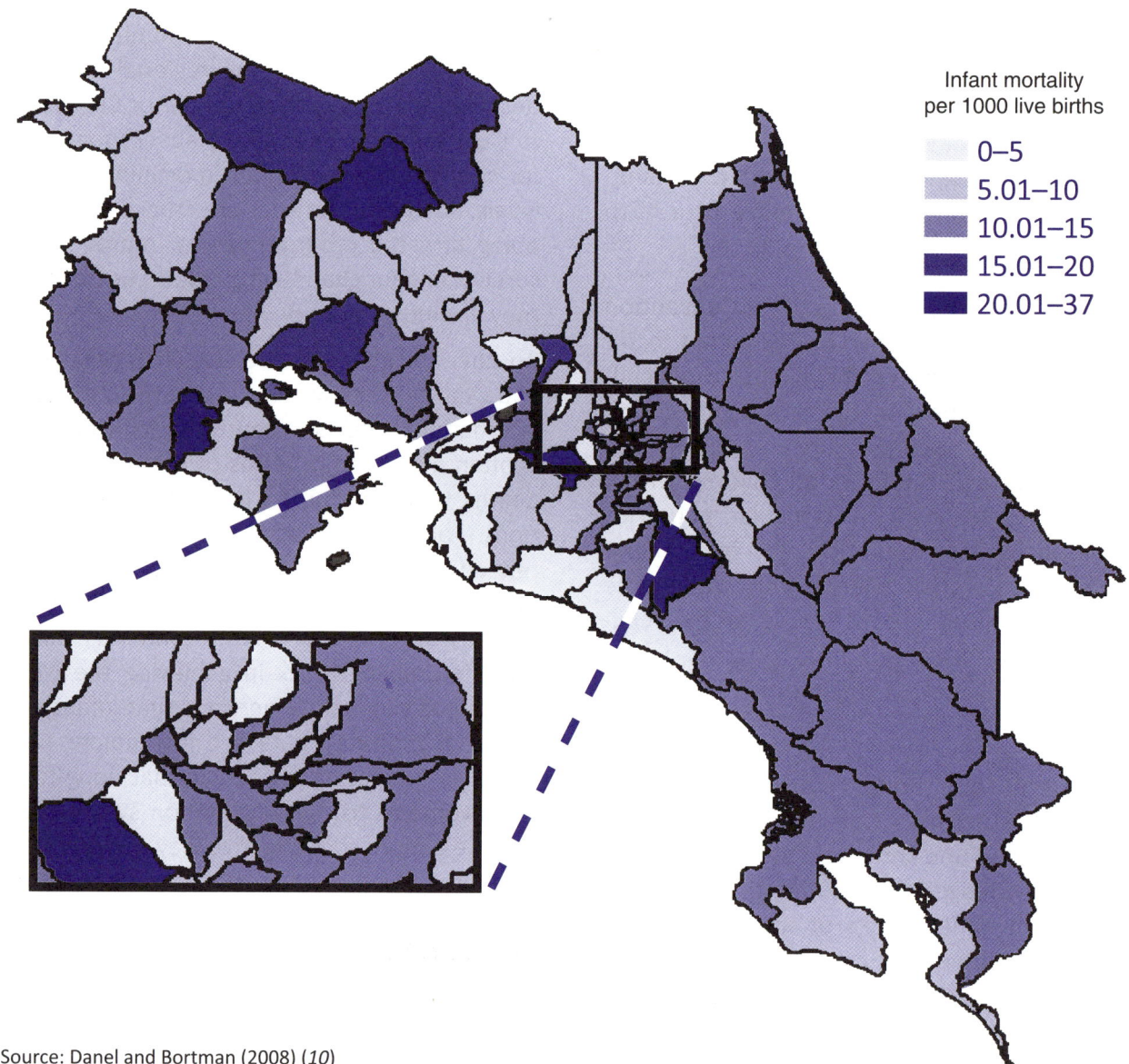

Source: Danel and Bortman (2008) (*10*)

(e.g. major noncommunicable diseases, injuries and violence) affect the population.

Several developing countries have used birth registration to identify geographical differences in fertility, and have subsequently been able to introduce family planning programmes in locations where they were most needed. Birth monitoring has also shed light on some of the negative ramifications of new medical technologies, particularly prenatal sex-selection (*11*). In many countries, registration data provide the starting point for conducting studies of deaths in women of reproductive age; civil registration is thus an essential tool for obtaining more effective estimates of the true extent of maternal mortality and generating an understanding of the underlying causes and circumstances.

The careful monitoring of vital statistics can effectively identify populations with excessive mortality, or those that urgently require specific programmes for disease control or health promotion. Vital statistics are the *only* empirical basis upon which annual progress can be monitored in a variety of public health programmes at subnational, national and global levels. In countries with well-developed systems, vital statistics have guided policy and prevention programmes, and have been used to support critical epidemiological research, ranging from ecological studies and descriptive epidemiology to studies of how occupational and genetic diseases affect different population groups.

1.6.3 Summary of uses and benefits

In many countries where birth and death registration is compulsory, laws also specify that annual statistics must be published (by sex and age) nationally and subnationally. Box 1.1 summarizes the many uses of vital statistics for human and social development.

1.7 Global status of civil registration and vital statistics systems

Neglect of civil registration systems has been called "the single most critical failure of development over the past 30 years" (*11*). Globally, information on vital statistics compares poorly with the detailed economic information available for most countries. Health information should be seen to be as important as economic data in supporting human development policies. Because of the absence of reliable vital statistics, many developing countries are now facing a rapid health transition but do not have reliable, timely and relevant information to guide the development of health priorities for their populations.

The global public health community, donors and development partners should support countries in their efforts to strengthen their civil registration and vital statistics systems. Given the efforts and expense that countries expend in maintaining civil registration systems, it is unacceptable to produce data that are biased, incomplete or out of date, and thus cannot be used for planning purposes. At the same time, national governments must acknowledge their responsibility for improving their systems, and must take the lead in efforts to register all births and deaths, and to medically certify all causes of deaths. It is in the interest of national governments and their citizens to ensure that civil registration systems count everyone – and make everyone count.

Despite the undoubted benefits of vital-events registration, only about one third of WHO member countries have systems that are considered to be essentially complete and to produce reliable data (*12*). In the other two thirds, many births and deaths are not registered, and information on the cause of death is often unreliable, if it is collected at all.

Box 1.1   Summary of uses of civil registration and vital statistics data

Individuals

Individuals use birth and death certificates issued by civil registration as evidence of:
- identity and age; for example, to apply for a passport, open bank accounts, access education and employment, protect ownership rights, access medical and social services, make insurance claims and conduct voting and other legal acts;
- origin and nationality when dealing with government or private business.

Local and national government authorities

Local and national government authorities use the birth and death registers derived from civil registration records to:
- calculate the number of citizens each year for administrative areas by age and sex;
- provide denominator data for calculating health-related indicators;
- make population projections for future planning;
- help to guide efficient resource allocation;
- carry out policy making at local levels for planning health, education services, housing, etc.;
- address health inequities from communicable disease, chronic disease and injuries;
- generate "life tables" and life expectancies for many health-planning purposes;
- measure progress on the MDGs and other international health goals;
- prepare polling lists for eligible voters for election purposes;
- calculate the number of members of parliament for each state or province;
- allocate budgets for development and for human resources.

Introduction

Figure 1.2 Quality of globally available information on causes of death

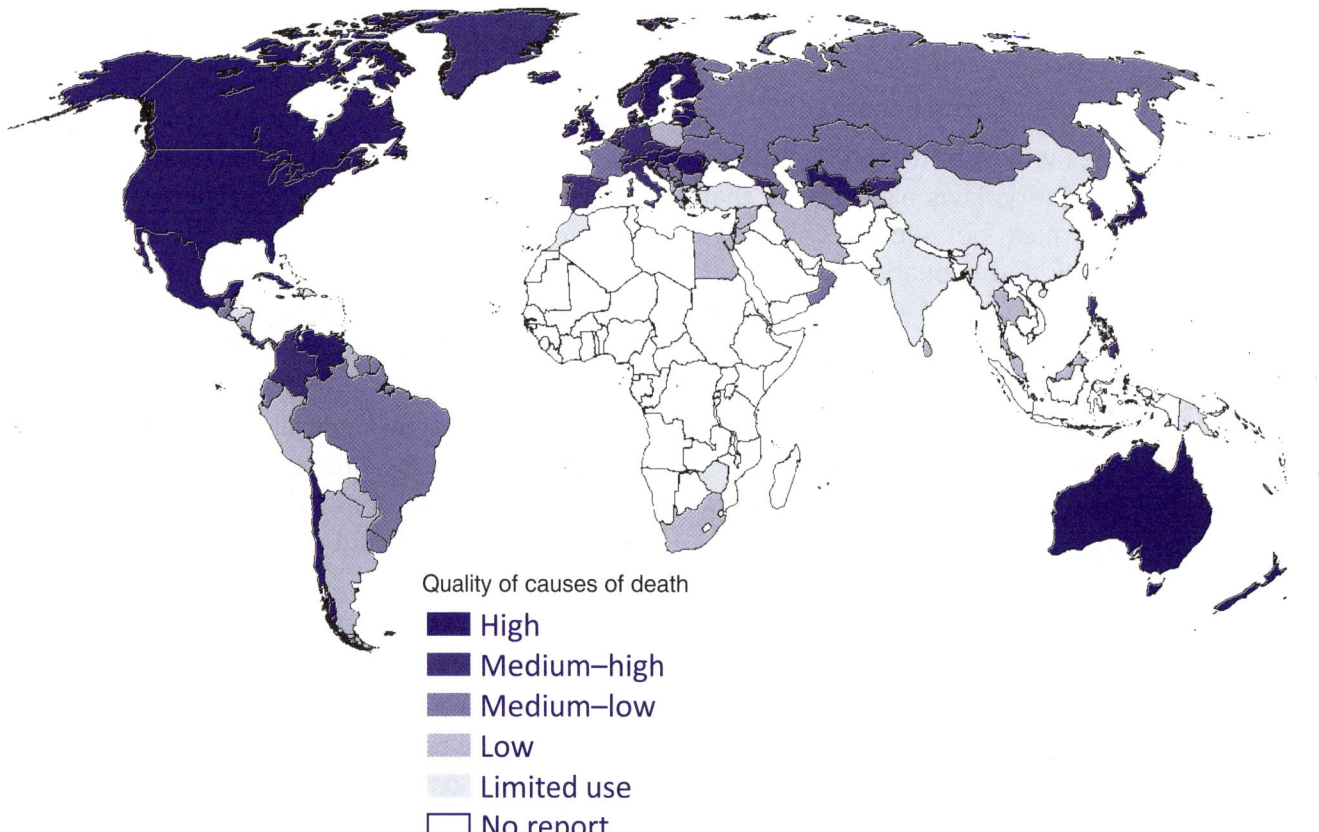

The boundaries and names shown and the designation used on this map do not imply the expression of any opinion whatsoever on the part of the WHO concerning the legal status of any country, territory, city or area of its authorities, or concerning the delimitation of its frontiers or boundaries.

Map production: Public Health Mapping and GIS Communicable Diseases (CDS), WHO.

© WHO 2007. All rights reserved.

2 Process for reviewing civil registration and vital statistics systems

This chapter provides a roadmap for using the WHO guidance tool to review and strengthen civil and vital statistics systems. The process has three phases:

- *Phase 1* – Leadership coordination and review (i.e. preparing for and carrying out the review);
- *Phase 2* – Priority setting and planning (i.e. developing a strategic plan for strengthening the system);
- *Phase 3* – Implementation (i.e. implementing the strategic plan).

These three phases are summarized in Box 2.1 and shown as a flowchart in Annex A. They align with the phases defined in the HMN document *Framework and standards for country health information systems* (*2*). Thus, countries can easily integrate the three phases into a more broadly based strategic development plan.

This document provides detailed guidance for Phases 1 and 2; less detail is provided for Phase 3 because this is likely to vary for each country, depending on national processes and the development environment. However, detailed information on strategic planning is given in the HMN document *Guidance for the health information systems (HIS) strategic planning process* (*13*).

Each country is free to adapt the suggested roadmap to their specific situation. However, adherence to the overall process is important because this will provide insights into how the civil registration and vital statistics systems function, which is necessary for improving those systems.

The roadmap lists only the main steps and the sequence recommended for a country to follow when undertaking a thorough review of its civil registration and vital statistics systems. Each country may add intermediate steps as necessary, to ensure that everyone involved clearly understands how to conduct the review and answer the assessment questions given in Chapter 3.

Sections 2.1–2.8, below, discuss the steps involved in Phases 1 and 2.

Box 2.1	Roadmap of actions and outcomes of the review	
Steps	Actions	Outcomes
Phase 1 — Leadership coordination and review		
1	Identify a lead agency that can initiate the process of forming a review committee; identify and invite stakeholders, and make a case to government of the need to improve the vital statistics system	■ Lead agency identified ■ Stakeholders identified and invited ■ Review committee formed ■ Case made to government
2	Undertake a rapid assessment of the current system, to build the case and prepare for the launch of the review	■ Rapid assessment undertaken by review committee ■ Meeting agenda developed
3	Conduct a launch meeting (to raise awareness, expand committee and form subgroups)	■ Stakeholders invited to launch meeting ■ Awareness raised among stakeholders of the need to improve vital statistics ■ Assessment framework and review process introduced to participants ■ Review committee expanded (if required) ■ Subgroups formed
4	Conduct an initial committee meeting (without subgroups)	■ Workplan and review schedule developed ■ Guidelines, and report template for subgroups, developed
5	Conduct review through subgroup work sessions	■ Review questions adapted ■ Detailed review of subcomponents produced ■ Subgroup reports with recommendations prepared for presentation to review committee

Process for reviewing civil registration and vital statistics systems

Box 2.1	Roadmap of actions and outcomes of the review (cont.)	
Steps	Actions	Outcomes
Phase 2 — Priority setting and planning		
6	Conduct a review committee results meeting with subgroups	■ Report presented and its recommendations collectively discussed ■ Recommendations for action agreed and prioritized ■ Case made to government
7	Conduct a review committee meeting or meetings without subgroups, to develop strategic plan	■ Strategic plan for improving the current vital statistics system prioritized and costed
8	Conduct a large stakeholder meeting to present improvement plan	■ Plan to strengthen the vital statistics system approved by wider stakeholder group
Phase 3 — Implementation		
There are no specific steps for this phase, because the process for achieving the various outcomes will vary by country		■ Resources allocated and finances mobilized ■ Implementation commenced ■ Monitoring commenced ■ Reprogramming undertaken as necessary

2.1 Phase 1: Step 1 – Form a review committee and raise awareness

2.1.1 Identify a lead agency

To start the process and form a review committee, it is necessary to first nominate an agency that can lead the review, and can identify and invite other stakeholders. In many settings, the initial impetus for this stage has come from one government agency, or from one or more committed individuals or country champions who are working in the area of health and vital statistics, and are eager to improve the availability and quality of vital statistics.

2.1.2 Form a review committee

Local participation

The review committee must have strong representation from all the ministries and departments involved in the collection, production and use of vital statistics. In general, at least 10 members will be needed to ensure that all key stakeholders are included. In some countries, an intergovernmental or interinstitutional committee of stakeholders may already have been established to coordinate the production of vital statistics. If such a committee does exist, it could form the core of the review committee.

The composition of the group will vary by country, but typically it would include:

- ■ staff from the following:
  - civil registration office;
  - ministry of health;
  - national statistics office;
  - office of the "registrar general" or similar office;
  - local government;
  - justice and planning authorities;
  - any other government departments responsible for collecting or using vital statistics;
- ■ other important stakeholders and users of the data (e.g. hospitals, public health institutions, medical associations and academia);
- ■ local representatives from UNICEF, UNFPA and WHO;
- ■ NGOs active in civil rights and birth registration (e.g. Plan International, World Vision and Save the Children).

Although the support of senior government officials is crucial for the success of the review, the actual process of evaluation is best carried out by those responsible for recording, compiling and analysing the data at national and subnational levels. These are likely to include mid-level statisticians from the national statistical office; officials working in the civil registration and vital statistics systems; and analysts, technical officers and practitioners in the health sector. Since the review will necessarily involve clinical judgement of the accuracy of cause-of-death diagnosis, medical doctors should form part of the team for specific tasks.

External assistance

Although this guidance tool has been developed for countries to use without external "technical assistance", some countries may find it helpful to draw on experts who can provide initial guidance to those involved in the review. For example, it may be helpful to engage a facilitator to:

- help launch the review process;
- explain the work to be carried out;
- meet with the people who will carry out the review;
- make sure that the review questions are fully understood.

Some facilitation may also be useful in reviewing the results. However, the effectiveness of the review will depend mainly on the active participation of all the main stakeholders, and their ability to build consensus around priority needs for improvement. Some countries request technical assistance from development agencies or international organizations for strengthening their health information systems. Such countries may wish to include cost estimates for the strengthening of various priority components, as identified by the review process.

2.1.3 Make a case to government

Before the review starts, the review committee may need to build awareness among senior government policy-makers, to gain their support. Given that civil registration is operated and funded by government authorities, high-level political commitment will be essential if the findings are to be implemented and improvements sustained. If the review committee feels that there is limited understanding of the importance of vital statistics, it should build awareness among key government personnel of the significance of reliable data on births, deaths and causes of death for policy and planning, as well as for health protection and promotion.

Civil society groups can be useful allies in drawing attention to the important human and civil rights aspects of civil registration. The review committee can engage these groups to help to mobilize stakeholders around the importance of good vital statistics for all sectors, not just health.

2.2 Step 2 – Undertake a rapid assessment

Before undertaking the detailed review, the review committee may find it useful to undertake a rapid assessment as a quick means of assessing the state of their current civil registration and vital statistics systems. The accompanying document – *Rapid assessment of national civil registration and vital statistics systems* – contains the rapid assessment tool, which was designed for that purpose and helps to highlight areas of weakness or concern. Although it provides a quick overview of how well or poorly a country's overall system is functioning, the rapid assessment tool is not a replacement for the detailed procedures outlined in this document. Rather, the committee can use the results from the rapid assessment to raise awareness and decide whether a full assessment using the detailed assessment tool is needed.

The rapid assessment tool consists of 25 questions, which are grouped into 11 areas that correspond to the main elements of the full assessment framework (Chapter 3). Each question in the rapid assessment allows countries to select one of four scenarios (labelled A–D) describing a typical range of hypothetical situations. A numeric value (0–3) is attached to each scenario, allowing a total score to be obtained. The total score will clearly indicate whether there is a need to carry out the detailed assessment.

The review committee or a core group of main stakeholders should carry out the rapid assessment, and scores should be given only after the group has discussed and reflected on the question. Scoring can be done either by reaching a consensus for each question and allocating a single score, or by individual group members

Process for reviewing civil registration and vital statistics systems

scoring each question (after the discussions); the scores should then be averaged to produce a final score for the question. Based on the total score obtained, the functioning of the national system can be rated. Table 2.1 shows the ratings for the range of possible scores, and outlines the action required for each rating.

All countries that score less than 85% on the rapid assessment are strongly advised to undertake a full assessment, and to produce and implement an improvement plan.

2.3 Step 3 – Launch the review

2.3.1 Launch meeting

If the review committee decides that, based on the evidence from the rapid assessment, the country should proceed to the detailed review, the committee needs to organize a launch meeting for the review. The meeting should have broad participation from all those involved in the collection, production and use of vital statistics – effective review depends on having all the main players represented at the launch and actively involved.

To get full collaboration of all key stakeholders, it is important that the launch meeting is carefully planned, with the review process well explained. Annex B provides a template for the agenda for the launch meeting.

The aims of the launch meeting are to:

- raise awareness of the importance of vital statistics and the need to improve the current system;
- get collaboration for undertaking the detailed review;
- inform stakeholders about the assessment framework and explain the review process;
- formalize the membership of the review committee;
- form subgroups to carry out the detailed review work.

2.3.2 Subgroups

The launch meeting can be used to expand the committee (if necessary) and to establish subgroups to conduct the technical aspects of the review according to the assessment framework given in Chapter 3. The number of subgroups needed and the allocation of tasks among them will vary; typically, 5–10 subgroups will be needed, as shown by the example in Box 2.2. The codes A1–E3, shown in parentheses in Box 2.2, represent the different subcomponents that make up the assessment framework (see Box 3.1). The whole framework is discussed in detail in Chapter 3.

Using the launch meeting to also decide on subgroups and tasks allows participants to elect to join a particular subgroup or suggest colleagues who might be invited to work with specific subgroups to provide necessary expertise. The criterion for participation in each subgroup should be expert knowledge of the topic to be reviewed. Group members should include, but not necessarily be limited to, representatives from the civil registration office (or other data collection agency), the ministry responsible for registration, the ministry of health and the national statistical office.

Table 2.1 Scores, ratings and actions required for rapid assessment

Score (%)	Rating	Actions required
<34	Dysfunctional	System requires substantial improvement in all areas
35–64	Weak	Many aspects of the system do not function well, and multiple issues require attention
65–84	Functional but inadequate	System works but some elements function poorly and require attention; specific weaknesses of the system should be identified by completing the comprehensive review
85–100	Satisfactory	Minor adjustments may be required in an otherwise well-functioning system

Process for reviewing civil registration and vital statistics systems

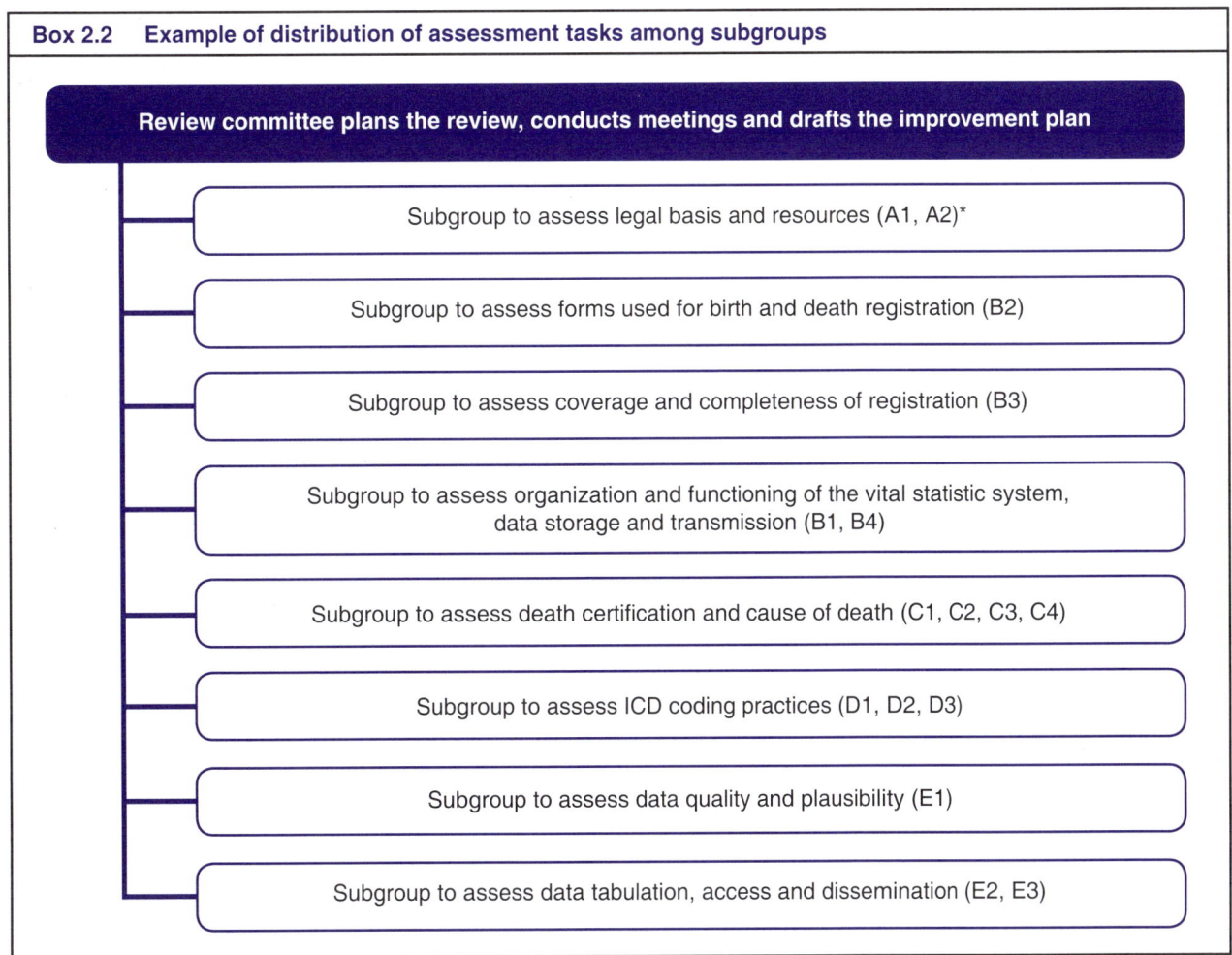

Box 2.2 Example of distribution of assessment tasks among subgroups

ICD, International statistical classification of diseases and related health problems

* The codes A1–E3 relate to the parts of the assessment framework summarized in Box 3.1 and discussed in full in Chapter 3.

2.4 Step 4 – Conduct an initial committee meeting

Following the launch meeting, the formalized review committee should meet, without the subgroups, to develop a workplan and a schedule for the work of the subgroups. The committee might also want to prepare some guidelines, or possibly a template outlining what the subgroups' reports should contain. This will facilitate the subgroups' work and be useful for the general discussion at the results meeting.

2.5 Step 5 – Conduct work sessions with subgroups

The final step in Phase 1 is for the subgroups to carry out detailed reviews of specific aspects of the civil registration and vital statistics systems, using the assessment framework given in Chapter 3. Each subgroup should be led by someone with sufficient expertise in the subject matter reviewed to guide the subgroup's discussion, and report the findings and recommendations to the review committee. A member of the review committee who is familiar with both the subject and the assessment framework would be suitable for this leadership task. Other possible leaders might be technical staff from the civil registration office, the national statistical office or the ministry of health, or experts with specific technical knowledge from universities or specialized institutions.

It is up to the identified leader to carefully study the review questions, and prepare a workplan for the subgroup. At the first subgroup meeting, it is recommended that the members review and adjust the questions suggested for assessing the specific area. Because of the wide variation in

Improving the quality and use of birth, death and cause-of-death information

the legal, organizational and technical aspects of different national civil registration and vital statistics systems, the assessment questions proposed for each component (presented in Chapter 3) cannot possibly cover every national situation.

The subgroups should meet as many times as required to complete the assigned tasks, and then prepare a report on their findings. The report should critically examine the issue or issues raised by the review question, and summarize the discussion for each question, as appropriate, rather than provide a simple response to the questions. For example, if the subgroup discussion reveals a problem or malfunction, the part of the report covering this question should contain:

- a concise statement of the problem, and suggestions for what needs to be improved or changed;
- specific benefits that could be expected from any improvements or changes;
- one or more specific recommendations for the changes required;
- specific suggestions for implementing the recommendations.

In other words, it is not sufficient to state that there is a problem – a potential solution for how to solve the problem also has to be provided. Having several subgroups working in parallel means that the groups can explore their specific areas in detail, without the process being too long or onerous. The country experiences seem to indicate that most subgroups will only need to meet a couple of times to complete their tasks.

2.6 Phase 2: Step 6 – Conduct a results meeting

Once the subgroups have prepared their reports, the first step in Phase 2 of the process is for the review committee to organize a results meeting where all the subgroups can present their findings and recommendations for improvement. The aim is to arrive at a set of agreed recommendations for priority activities covering the entire civil registration and vital statistics systems.

Once all the subgroups have presented their findings, and these have been thoroughly discussed and reviewed by the meeting, the recommendations that are retained will need to be prioritized. This can be done at the end of the meeting, by listing all the recommendations and scoring them as high, medium or low priority, according to appropriate criteria. The review committee could suggest some criteria during the discussion of the recommendations, and allow meeting participants to jointly score all the recommendations. Criteria might include the following:

- *Urgency* – Is the activity of such critical importance for subsequent activities in the vital statistics strengthening plan that it needs to be addressed immediately, or can it be delayed for a defined period (e.g. 12 months or longer)?
- *Feasibility* – How easily can the activity be implemented? Does it require interdepartmental agreement, high-level approval or even a change in legislation?
- *Cost* – What are the cost implications? Can the activity be funded within the existing budget or is additional funding necessary?
- *Time* – How long will it take to complete the activity?

The outcome of the meeting should be a list of agreed and prioritized recommendations, which will form the core of an improvement plan for the country's civil registration and vital statistics systems.

2.7 Step 7 – Conduct a review committee meeting to draft a strategic plan

Shortly after the results meeting, the review committee needs to meet, to complete the details of the rough suggestions for improvement agreed on at the results meeting with the subgroups. The aim of this meeting is to begin drafting a detailed strategic plan for improving the civil registration and vital statistics systems, with costs estimates, a time schedule and clear responsibilities assigned to each stakeholder for implementing the actions. The committee should also discuss whether there is a need for technical assistance for specific tasks, and whether funding from external donors will be required for some of the actions.

2.8 Step 8 – Conduct a final stakeholder meeting

As soon as the review committee has prepared the strategic improvement plan, a final meeting should be organized so that the plan can be presented to a broad range of stakeholders, including international organizations and donors. The aim of this meeting should be to gain broad approval and support for the strategic plan, so that implementation of improvements to the current vital statistics system can begin.

2.9 Phase 3 – Implementation

As explained above, no detailed guidance is given in the current report for this phase, because the specific actions and the way the strategic plan is implemented will vary among countries. However, some issues are common to implementing the findings of the review, and these are briefly discussed here.

2.9.1 Towards sustainable civil registration and vital statistics systems

For all countries, civil registration is a long-term investment and, unlike ad hoc surveys, it needs to be continually maintained; this has to be reflected in both the strategic plan (which should span at least 5–10 years) and the implementation of the improvements (which should be stepwise). Collecting and producing vital statistics typically involves many departments; therefore, maintenance and development costs can be shared. The information generated will support not only vital statistics, but also other government functions such as legal documentation, electoral rolls, population projections and health-outcome monitoring.

Local authorities are key players in the implementation of the changes; thus, they need to be convinced that birth and death certification is an indispensable aspect of citizenship and governance, and that births and deaths need to be properly recorded. In countries where government processes are decentralized, there is likely to be a strong demand for local vital statistics information for planning purposes, and this should be carefully catered for in the implementation. However, for data to be useful at the national level, a standardized approach to collecting the vital event information is needed; hence, it is necessary to have careful central management of implementation of the changes.

Countries that are at the early stages of building civil registration and vital statistics systems need to be aware that fully functioning and complete systems take time to establish. Nevertheless, it is possible to make steady progress on both access to, and completeness of, civil registration and vital statistics if it is fully integrated into the development process. In countries where registration offices and infrastructure are lacking, schools and primary health-care facilities could be used as interim registration points until the government has the resources to extend the registration infrastructure.

2.9.2 Monitoring progress

As part of the implementation of the improvement plan, countries need to monitor their progress by periodically assessing their civil registration and vital statistics systems. This regular monitoring of progress in the development plan does not need to be onerous, and this guidance tool proposes a few performance indicators to measure progress every 3–4 years. For example, vital statistics systems can be evaluated in relation to coverage, completeness, data quality (accuracy and relevance), timeliness of the data and how the data is used; and civil registration systems can be evaluated in terms of their functioning. Annex C contains further suggestions for indicators that can be used to periodically assess progress. Countries can, of course, select other indicators that better reflect the development status of their particular systems.

3 The WHO assessment framework

This chapter describes the WHO assessment framework that the subgroups will use in undertaking a detailed review of a country's civil registration and vital statistics systems. It explains how the framework was developed and is structured, and outlines the various components and subcomponents.

3.1 Development and structure

The WHO assessment framework builds on previous research on vital statistics, notably on various assessment frameworks and indicators (*4, 12, 14–17*). It has also been informed by the experience of several contributors involved in conducting empirical assessments in countries in different regions of the world. For example, PAHO developed a questionnaire to collect information from their member countries on vital statistics, morbidity and health resources (*18*). Many Latin American countries are familiar with the PAHO questionnaire. Specifically, the questionnaire collected information about the general organization of the vital statistics systems in member countries, procedures for data production at various levels and reasons for data incompleteness. Application of the questionnaire provided background material for a regional plan of action for strengthening vital and health statistics in the PAHO region.

The WHO assessment framework has hugely benefited from the UN guidelines and recommendations on the establishment and operation of civil registration and vital statistics systems, and is fully aligned with these guidelines and recommendations (*1, 19–22*).

Most previous research has concentrated on assessing the coverage or completeness of the data produced. This framework goes further by evaluating issues related to the functioning of the system that produces the data, and hence diagnosing potential problem areas. The rationale for this approach is that the way the subsystems function determines the reliability and completeness of the data produced. In other words, the inputs and processes of the civil registration and vital statistics systems need to be fully understood if lasting improvements are to be made to the output. All three aspects – inputs, processes and outputs – are therefore crucial to the functioning of a vital statistics system, and should be part of any in-depth review.

Both the HMN *Framework and standards for country health information systems* (*2*) and its associated tool *Assessing the national health information system* (*23*) briefly discuss vital statistics and civil registration. However, the approach used in this guidance tool, although in line with these documents, is much more detailed and comprehensive.

3.2 Overview of components and subcomponents of the WHO assessment framework

The framework consists of five key components (A–E) of the civil registration and vital statistics systems. It comprehensively covers inputs, processes and outputs from these components, as shown in Table 3.1.

Table 3.1 Inputs, processes and outputs

Aspect	Components	Areas covered
Inputs	A	■ Legislative and regulatory frameworks supporting the existence and operation of civil registration and vital statistics systems, as well as the financial, human and technological resources required for proper functioning of civil registration and vital statistics systems
Processes	B–D	■ Processes required for obtaining and compiling information such as registration and certification practices ■ Forms, classifications and coding practices used in obtaining and compiling information ■ Procedures for the management and transmission of data
Outputs	E	■ Type and quality of statistics produced, and methods for disseminating, accessing and using those statistics

Improving the quality and use of birth, death and cause-of-death information 17

The WHO assessment framework

Details of the assessment framework are shown in Box 3.1, with components A–E broken down into 16 subcomponents (A1–E3). The sections that follow explain each subcomponent by discussing and investigating specific questions and issues. Any preparatory work needed to facilitate the discussion and review is highlighted at the beginning of the subcomponent. Also, where required, further explanation and guidance are provided for specific review questions, to give additional context or to highlight important items.

3.3 Component A – Legal basis and resources for civil registration

This section covers component A – *Legal basis and resources for civil registration* – within which are the following subcomponents:

- A1 – National legal framework for civil registration and vital statistics systems;
- A2 – Registration infrastructure and resources.

Vital statistics are derived from records collected through the civil registration system, which needs to be anchored in a sound legal and regulatory framework. Legislation is essential to:

- ensure the universality and continuity of the civil registration system;
- ensure the regular dissemination of data and the confidentiality of individual information;
- clarify the functions and responsibilities of the different government agencies involved.

A national civil registration Act or similar is therefore a fundamental requirement for a sustainable and functioning civil registration system. The Act must be associated with rules and regulations that specify:

- what information is to be collected, by whom, from whom and by when;
- who is responsible for compiling the information and transforming it into statistics;

Box 3.1	WHO assessment framework
Inputs **A**	**Legal basis and resources for civil registration** ■ **A1** – National legal framework for civil registration and vital statistics systems ■ **A2** – Registration infrastructure and resources
Processes **B**	**Registration practices, coverage and completeness** ■ **B1** – Organization and functioning of the civil registration and vital statistics systems ■ **B2** – Review of forms used for birth and death registration ■ **B3** – Coverage and "completeness of registration" ■ **B4** – Data storage and transmission
C	**Death certification and cause of death** ■ **C1** – ICD-compliant practices for death certification (*24*) ■ **C2** – Hospital death certification ■ **C3** – Deaths occurring outside hospital ■ **C4** – Practices affecting the quality of cause-of-death data
D	**ICD mortality coding practices** ■ **D1** – Mortality coding practices ■ **D2** – Mortality coder qualification and training ■ **D3** – Quality of mortality coding
Outputs **E**	**Data access, use and quality checks** ■ **E1** – Data quality and plausibility checks ■ **E2** – Data tabulation ■ **E3** – Data access and dissemination

- who is tasked with management and dissemination of the data.

Although most countries have a civil registration Act or similar legislation, it is often outdated, does not cover key aspects, or is poorly complied with because it is not enforced.[2]

Legal systems and practices vary from country to country, which means that legislation will also vary. However, the basic statutes should be similar and should, if possible, align with UN principles and international standards for civil registration and vital statistics (1, 22). The UN Statistics Division has a mandate to help countries to strengthen their civil registration and vital statistics systems, and it has considerable experience in providing guidance to countries on the legal, organizational and technical aspects of such systems.

The UN guidelines for establishing the legal basis for civil registration were prepared more than 10 years ago. Nevertheless, they continue to be useful to countries in strengthening their legal frameworks and developing relevant regulations covering all important aspects of a national civil registration system, including its statistical function. The guidance given here closely adheres to the advice and standards provided in the UN handbook on preparing a legal framework for civil registration (21).[3]

To function effectively, civil registration systems also depend on adequate annual budgets from government, to pay staff and to create and maintain sufficient registration facilities. Other prerequisites are the availability of trained staff to register events and compile the data into statistics, and the tools and supplies they need to carry out their work. For computerized systems, budgets for equipment, maintenance and continuing staff training are also important.

Subcomponents A1 and A2, both of which are given in detail in the boxes below, cover the most pertinent issues to be assessed within this component. Each country that undertakes a detailed review must decide on the relevance of all the questions, and whether additional questions need to be included. By investigating each question or issue raised, a list of weaknesses in the national legal framework for civil registration and vital statistics can be generated, and agreement reached on the main issues requiring attention. Ensuring that appropriate legislation is in place is a critical first step in the overall plan for strengthening a country's civil registration system.

The system that produces vital statistics from civil registration can be configured in many ways, and responsibility for collecting, processing and maintaining the data varies from country to country. Depending on structures and traditions in countries, the national civil registration system may be centralized and operated by a single agency responsible for issuing certificates and coordinating all registration efforts at the national level. Alternatively, the system may be decentralized, with individual states or administrative areas responsible for the registration of the vital events in their areas. The legal framework needs to reflect the national system of birth and death registration in place, the local practices for certifying deaths and disposing of deceased persons, the method by which the information is compiled into vital statistics and who is responsible for disseminating them.

A common structure in many countries is that a registrar general or similar high-level official in the civil registration (located in the ministry of interior or another ministry with similar responsibilities) is responsible for the national registration of vital events. Whether the organizational structure is centralized or decentralized, birth and death information is collected through a network of local area registration offices that are supported in their functions by other reporting units such as the police, hospitals, health clinics, mortuaries and community leaders. The compilation of the collected information and its transformation into vital statistics is often delegated to the national statistical office, which might

---

[2]This is confirmed by the *Country health information system assessment* reports posted on the HMN web site: http://www.who.int/healthmetrics/support/en/

[3]An example of a comprehensive, organic civil registration law with custom-designed legislation (and sample forms) can be found in the United Nations handbook, pp. 144–208. http://unstats.un.org/unsd/publication/SeriesF/SeriesF_71E.pdf

The WHO assessment framework

receive technical support from the ministry of health for coding and processing the cause-of-death data. Figure 3.1 illustrates such a system (this is an idealized example because it assumes that all births and deaths are registered).

In many cases, there is close coordination between all the government agencies involved, but coordination can sometimes be a major challenge. Some countries may even run dual systems: one that is concerned only with registration, and that issues birth and death certificates to individuals; and another that collects vital statistics through the health system. Dual data collection systems are prevalent in Latin America in particular, and the operation and division of responsibility in such systems needs to be considered carefully to avoid unnecessary duplication and inconsistencies in the reported numbers of births and deaths.

Civil registration systems need adequate resources to support the required functions, including registration of events, and retrieving and archiving of records. Similarly, the agency that is mandated with preparing the vital statistics from birth and death records requires adequate resources to collect the data from local registration points, and to clean, store and collate the information in ways that allow useful dissemination. These agencies need to employ and teach staff to carry out tasks; also, they incur maintenance costs and investment expenses when introducing new technologies and educating staff in their operation. The budget needed to finance fully functioning civil registration and vital statistics systems will vary according to prevailing levels of system development, but it will always be significant.

As discussed in Chapter 1, there are costs associated with *not* having good vital statistics; these appear in the form of misallocated resources, and misguided policies and programs that are based on wrong information. In addition, any intermediary alternatives to a vital statistics system, such as surveys and sample registration systems, will be costly to implement and maintain.

Figure 3.1 Schematic representation of civil registration and vital statistics systems

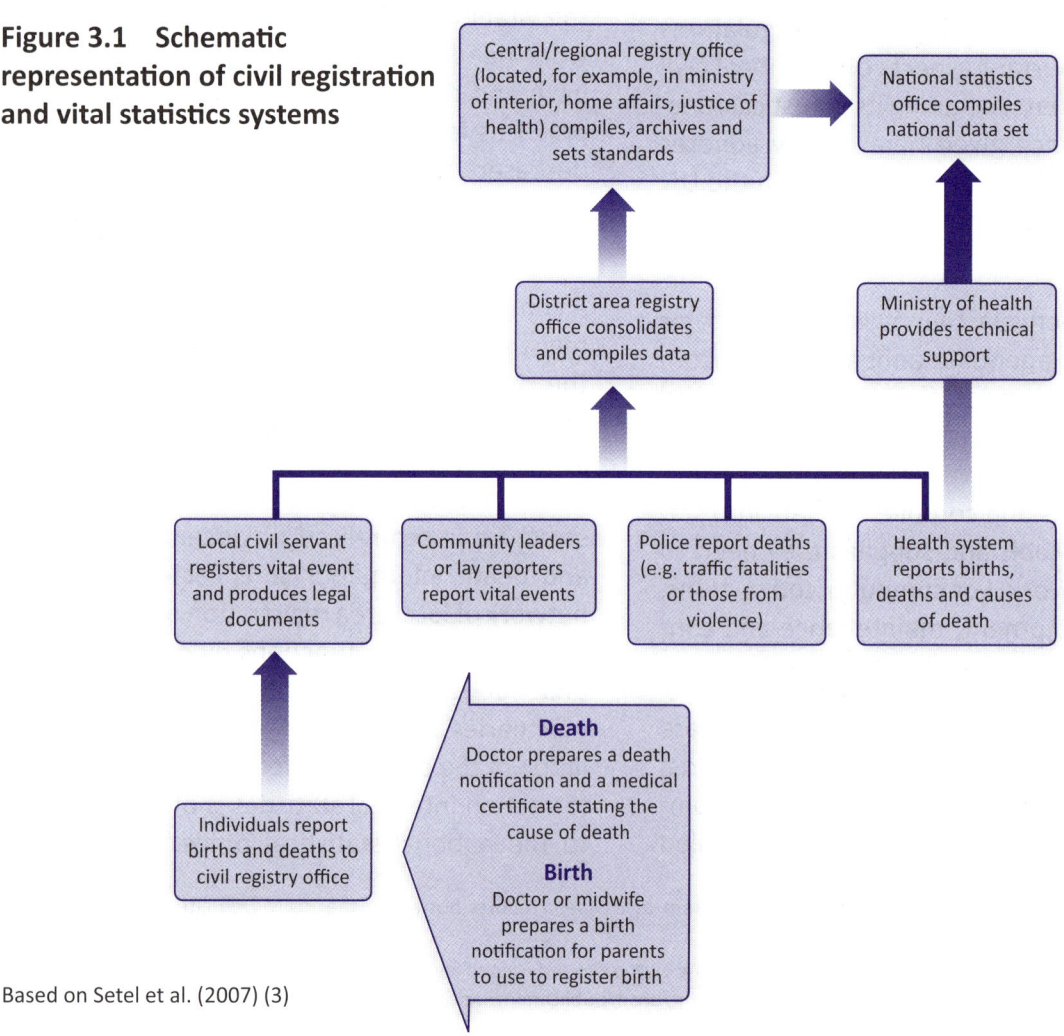

Based on Setel et al. (2007) (3)

20 *Improving the quality and use of birth, death and cause-of-death information*

The WHO assessment framework

Subcomponent A1: National legal framework for civil registration and vital statistics systems

Supporting material to be prepared in advance:

- Diagram that describes in detail the entire civil registration and vital statistics systems currently used in the country (see Figure 3.1 for an example).
- Inventory of all legal instruments (laws, rules and regulations) regarding civil registration and vital statistics, including relevant regulation concerning cemeteries, funeral parlours, sanitation (i.e. transportation and disposal of cadavers) and hospitals. Indicate the year each law or regulation was implemented. Briefly describe in lay terms the key elements of the law or regulation (this may be done by someone with legal experience from the registrar general's office).

The subgroup will use this material when discussing the questions and issues below on the laws and regulations governing the civil registration and vital statistics systems.

Civil registration is the system with which a government records the vital events of its citizens. The primary purpose of civil registration is to create legal documents that are used to establish and protect the civil rights of individuals.

A secondary purpose is to create data for the compilation of vital statistics. The system that uses the records for deriving statistics on vital events and the relevant characteristics of the events is referred to as the *vital statistics system*.

- **A1.1** Does the country have a law defining a civil registration system?
- **A1.2** Does the country have a law defining a vital statistics system?

To be useful, vital statistics should be derived from universal and continuous registration. By explicitly stating that registration is compulsory, and laying down penalties for non-registration, the law supports the registration of vital events. While timely registration should be encouraged, the penalty for registering older children should be low so that it does not constitute a barrier to "delayed registration".

- **A1.3** Does the law clearly state that birth and death registration is compulsory?
- **A1.4** Is there a penalty for non-registration of:
  - births?
  - deaths?
- **A1.5** If yes, please indicate the nature of the penalty.
  If there is a financial penalty, specify the current amount.
- **A1.6** Is the penalty routinely applied?

The WHO and the UN have agreed on definitions for what constitutes a live birth and a "stillbirth". These definitions have been included in the Glossary and, if not already given, should be introduced.

- **A1.7** Does the birth registration law give clear and unambiguous definitions to be used for:
  - live birth?
  - fetal death or stillbirth?
- **A1.8** Are these definitions aligned with the international standards in the Glossary?

The responsibility for registering birth usually falls on a parent. Usually, the birth attendant or institution where the birth took place must write a birth "notification" that parents use to register the child, and sometimes must also report the birth to an official authority. For death, responsibility for registration falls on a near relative of the deceased. The reporting is the responsibility of the attending or family doctor or, if there was no witness to the death, the person who found the body of the deceased person.

- **A1.9** Is it stated in law who is responsible for registering births or deaths and who should declare or report births or deaths?
- **A1.10** If yes, provide details of all possible informants.

Improving the quality and use of birth, death and cause-of-death information

The WHO assessment framework

Subcomponent A1: National legal framework for civil registration and vital statistics systems (cont.)

When a vital event takes place in a health facility, the facility is often required to report it. Such facility-reported data can be used to verify the registration figures.

In many countries, the private sector is a significant provider of health care; hence, a substantial proportion of births and deaths occur in nongovernmental institutions. The law should require all of these institutions to report vital events.

A1.11 Is there a law or regulation requiring hospitals and health facilities to report births and deaths? If so, to what authorities do they report the births and deaths?

A1.12 If yes, to what authorities do they report the births and deaths?

A1.13 Does the law or regulation cover the private sector?
Does the law or regulation also include social security and other nongovernmental facilities?

The period within which the vital event must be reported must be specified in the civil registration law. This period may vary between countries, but should be consistent throughout the country. A shorter notification period is better than a longer one.

A1.14 Does the law state the time within which births and deaths should be registered?

A1.15 If yes, how long is the reporting period?

A1.16 Is the reporting period suitable and is it respected throughout the country?

Most countries have a grace period of one year within which "late registrations" are accepted before penalties apply. The law should make specific provision for the handling of late and delayed registration of vital events. Every effort should be made to avoid delayed registration.

A1.17 Does the law make provision for:
- late registration?
- delayed registration?

A1.18 Are there clear procedures for dealing with these cases?

Most countries have adopted the place of occurrence of the birth or death as the place for registration, but also request information about "usual residence" so that birth and death statistics can be compiled in both ways, according to intended use.

A1.19 Is it stated where births or deaths should be registered; for example, according to place of occurrence or place of usual residence?

The best way to avoid unnecessary duplication and ensure good collaboration is to have clarity in the law concerning the duties of each government department involved. The diagram of the civil and vital statistics systems prepared for discussion of this question can be used to examine the role of each government agency or office.

A1.20 Does the law clearly designate the functions, duties and responsibilities of each government department involved?

Registration of vital events should be free; hence, the cost of registration needs to be funded by government (national or local) budgetary allocations. This should be stated in law. The continuity of the registration process is a necessary part of producing useful outputs, and requires an agency with sufficient administrative stability and an appropriate annual budget allocation.

A1.21 Does the law establish how the civil registration and vital statistics systems are to be funded?

A1.22 Does the law stipulate that registration should be free of charge for all?

A1.23 If registration is not free, what is the fee to register:
- a birth?
- a death?

The WHO assessment framework

Subcomponent A1: National legal framework for civil registration and vital statistics systems (cont.)

It is generally in the interest of both the country and individuals for *all* the population to be registered, including citizens living abroad or displaced, and foreign nationals (including refugees and asylum seekers living in the country). However, it may be helpful to identify these groups separately for some uses of the data.

- **A1.24** Is the population covered by civil registration laws clearly defined? Is it, for example:
  - the entire population living in the country?
  - only citizens living in the country?
  - some other subsets of the population?
- **A1.25** What does the law require in relation to registering births and deaths of citizens living abroad?
- **A1.26** What does the law require in relation to registration of births and deaths of:
  - foreign nationals living in the country?
  - nomadic or displaced populations?
  - refugees and asylum seekers?

The confidentiality of the information provided in the individual records must be protected. The law must state who can access the information and for what purposes, in a way that protects confidential information from misuse.

- **A1.27** Does the law include confidentiality measures to protect individuals?
- **A1.28** Is it specified who can obtain copies of a person's birth and death certificates?

For public health purposes, medical certification of the cause of death is essential, because without it there will be little confidence in the accuracy of statistics on causes of death. In countries where many births and deaths take place at home, non-medically trained persons are given the task of certifying cause of death. However, there is limited public health value in non-medically certified data on causes of death.

- **A1.29** Does the law state who can certify death and the cause of death?

Many countries have laws referring to the disposal of bodies. An effective way to ensure that deaths are registered is to require death registration documents *before* burial or cremation can take place. Indeed, often it is the undertaker who is responsible for the registration, in which case the undertaker, with the assistance of relatives, prepares all the papers necessary for death registration, and must file these with the civil registration office before the deceased person can be transported to a final resting place.

- **A1.30** Does the law specify the official document(s) needed before a burial or cremation can take place?

Improving the quality and use of birth, death and cause-of-death information

The WHO assessment framework

Subcomponent A2: Registration infrastructure and resources

Supporting material to be prepared in advance:
- Map showing the location of all civil registration offices in the country and the administrative areas they cover. Indicate separately all other points of registration (e.g. hospitals or local registrars).
- Current budget allocations for civil registration functions at all levels of government, where available. (If these are unavailable, use estimates).

The civil registration budget should include all annual costs such as salaries and social contributions, maintenance of buildings and equipment, electricity and other running costs, and staff training and supplies. If the cost of the vital statistics system is included in the same budget, it should be indicated separately. Both the actual cost (or estimate) and a per capita figure should be provided for discussion.

- A2.1 What is the annual national operating budget for civil registration?
- A2.2 Can this budget be separately identified at state and municipal levels?
  Can the budgets for national, state and municipal levels be separately identified?

It is important to debate whether the annual funds allocated for operation of the vital statistics and civil registration systems are adequate. In this context, adequate means sufficient to carry out the intended functions within specified time limits and to the satisfaction of users, particularly government planning departments.

- A2.3 Are these funds adequate to ensure the proper functioning of the system?
- A2.4 Where would additional funding be likely to make the most difference?

Local "civil registrars" are people authorized to record vital events, irrespective of whether they are civil servants or are carrying out this function under another status rather than as their primary function.

- A2.5 How many local civil registrars does the country currently have?
- A2.6 Are they paid by:
  - central government?
  - local government?
  - fee-for-service?
  - other source?
- A2.7 Are there local variations in the way, and amounts, that registrars are paid? Explain these variations.

The most commonly reported obstacle to registration is that the registration office is too far away. Integrating registration points into hospitals is an effective way to improve the number of registrations. The map prepared for discussion of this question – showing the location of local civil registration offices and subsidiary registration units – can be used to respond to the following questions.

- A2.8 Are the number and distribution of local civil registration offices or registration points sufficient to cover the whole country?
- A2.9 Are there subsidiary reporting or registration units, such as hospitals or village officials, with registration duties?
- A2.10 Is there access to registration 24 hours a day, 7 days a week?

If poor access to civil registration points appears to contribute to low registration coverage, discuss whether mobile registration facilities would be useful or effective. In several countries, such registration outreach has improved civil registration among remote and hard-to-reach sectors of the population.

- A2.11 Are mobile registration facilities operational in remote or underserviced areas?
- A2.12 If yes, how many? Is the number of mobile registration services sufficient?
- A2.13 Is there a separate budget for registration outreach?

Subcomponent A2: Registration infrastructure and resources (cont.)

If an overall national registration development plan and continuous coverage of all regions are lacking, it will be difficult to lobby for additional funds for full coverage. Discuss possible approaches to achieving better coverage of birth and death registration, including the use of other public facilities such as schools and health clinics.

A2.14 Is there a national plan for achieving complete coverage of the country with registration offices or registration points?

A2.15 Over what period does this plan extend?

Based on the structure of the civil registration system, a matrix should be prepared, with the rows being the types of registration facility (e.g. urban office, rural and remote registration facility) and the columns the types of equipment. Respond to the following question separately for each equipment category.

A2.16 For each type of civil registration point, describe the technical equipment available in all or most offices; for example, telephones, photocopiers, scanners, computers and internet.

Training materials and published standards are crucial to ensure that all vital events are registered in the same way, irrespective of the office and person registering the event. Poorly trained or poorly motivated staff are less likely to help improve data quality at the critical point of data collection. Staff training with an adequate budget is essential, especially when new registration procedures are introduced.

A2.17 How are civil registrars selected?

A2.18 What qualifications do civil registrars need?

A2.19 Is there a budget for training civil registrars and staff involved in registration?

A2.20 Is there a budget for preparing and disseminating written training materials, such as handbooks on civil registration?

In most countries, official vital statistics are produced by a unit that is separate from the civil registration office; often, this unit is located in the national statistical office or ministry of health. In this case, there is usually a separate budget for producing and disseminating vital statistics that includes staff-related costs, office and equipment maintenance, supplies, dissemination costs and staff training.

A2.21 What is the current budget for the vital statistics unit? (If more than one office is involved, estimate a figure that covers all the vital statistics being compiled, including cause of death data.)

3.4 Component B – Registration practices, coverage and completeness

This section covers component B – *Registration practices, coverage and completeness* – within which are the following subcomponents:

- B1 – Organization and functioning of the civil registration and vital statistics systems;
- B2 – Review of forms used for birth and death registration;
- B3 – Coverage and completeness of registration;
- B4 – Data storage and transmission.

Component B is a process component of the assessment framework. It investigates:

- the systems in place to collect information on vital events and produce vital statistics;
- the kind of information collected;
- how data flow between different parts of the system;
- the completeness of registration data and vital statistics;
- the constraints in the system, and in society more generally, to improving the completeness of registration.

There are many steps between when a birth or death occurs and when it is included in a country's vital statistics. Timeliness of data depends not only on how quickly an event is registered, but also on how quickly the information is processed and forwarded to the vital statistics agency. Understanding what data are collected from individuals, and how they are transcribed, compiled, transmitted, checked and stored in archives and databases before becoming vital statistics, will help to identify potential problem areas in the system. This knowledge is also essential for understanding how to alleviate problems and improve the quality of the information produced.

This component also reviews how tasks are distributed between the civil registration authorities, the health system and the national statistical office (or any other institution involved), and how these parties cooperate. Areas of duplication – for example, collection tasks or maintenance of databases – are likely to be inefficient and should be carefully investigated, to ascertain whether they can be eliminated through improved collaboration.

To identify bottlenecks or loopholes, all operational procedures should be discussed in detail, starting from the occurrence of the events – births, deaths and fetal deaths (if recorded) – through all the steps in the entire registration process. This should be done separately for events that take place outside of hospitals and for those that occur within hospitals (both public and private). If special procedures exist for certifying accidental deaths (e.g. reporting to a coroner or similar), the procedures for registering these events should also be described and discussed.

There is an important distinction between notification of a death and certification of cause of death by a doctor. Responsibility for these two functions generally lies with the attending doctor, or with the family doctor if the death occurred at home. For births, it is the birth attendant who usually issues a birth notification. However, in most developing countries, the responsibility for registering births and deaths lies with the family, who may not understand the difference between the notification form completed by the doctor and the legal registration paper, and thus may not go to the civil registration office to register the event. In contrast, in many developed countries, the onus for registration is on the hospital, health institution or undertaker, and official registration papers are completed before the release of the body or before the baby leaves the institution. Whatever practice is followed, it must be described in sufficient detail to highlight deficiencies and obstacles in the birth and death registration processes.

The WHO assessment framework

In countries where the onus is on individuals and families to register births and deaths, it is important to ensure that registration procedures are not burdensome. To investigate how difficult and time-consuming the registration of a birth or death is, a small team (2–3 members) from the subgroup should try to gather information from a selection of registration offices of different sizes (including some operating outside major cities) about the following aspects of the registration process:

- How long does it take to complete a birth or death registration?
- Is the guidance given sufficient?
- Are citizens satisfied with the service?
- What problems do registration staff encounter in attempting to properly register births and deaths?

In some settings, deaths that are certified in hospitals can escape registration if it is possible to bury or cremate a body without a disposal permit from the civil registration authorities. This occurs with death registration and certification processes in Mexico (Figure 3.2). Similarly, although more than 90% of births in Mexico take place in medical establishments and are thus certified, families sometimes do not register the birth at the civil registration office (Figure 3.3). Failure to register a birth is likely to be more common for births occurring outside medical establishments, particularly if the baby dies shortly after birth. Countries should ensure that appropriate mechanisms are in place to eliminate or at least minimize the possibility of non-registration of both the birth and the death of infants who die shortly after birth. This information is critical for guiding policies to reduce infant mortality and improve child health services.

Figure 3.2 Death registration and certification process in Mexico

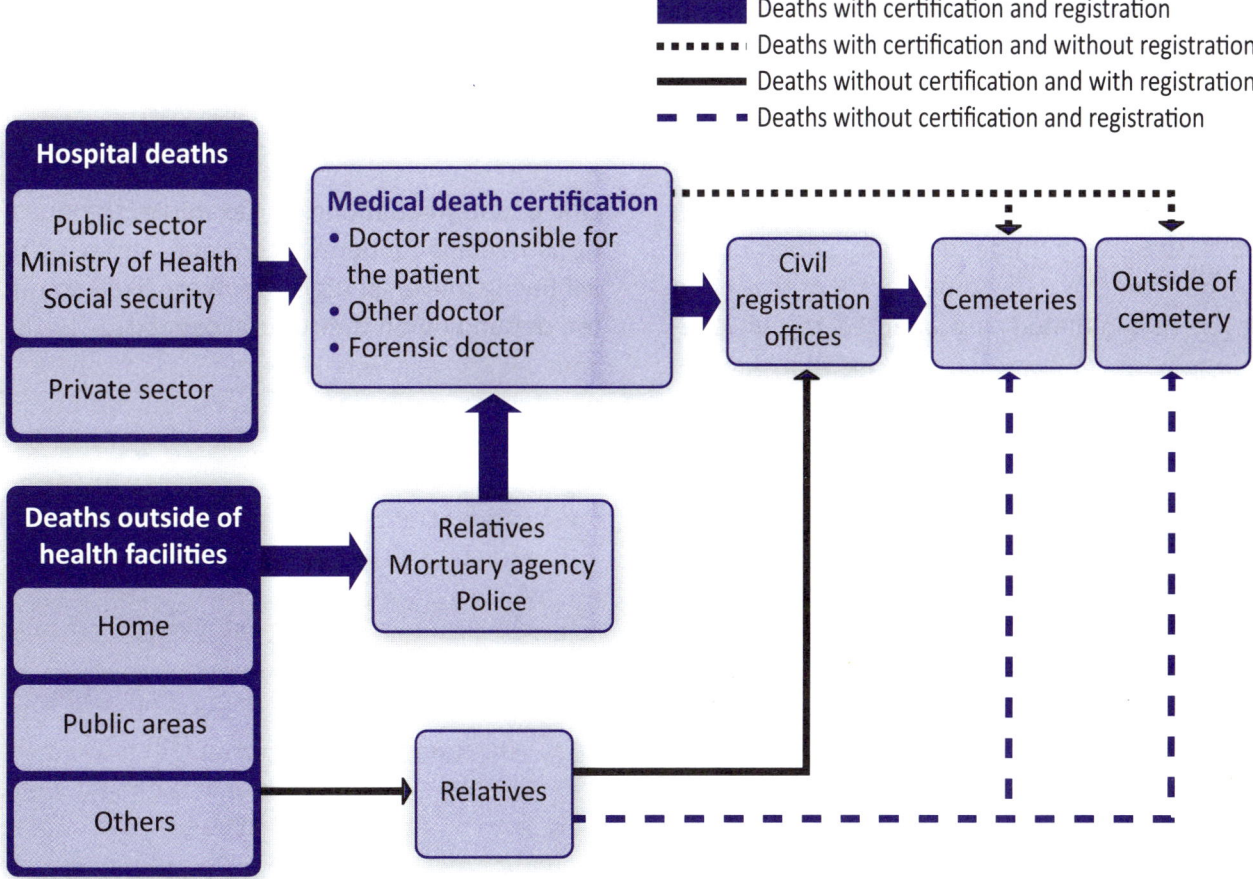

Source: R Lozano, Institute for Health Metrics and Evaluation, University of Washington, personal communication, 2009

Improving the quality and use of birth, death and cause-of-death information 27

The WHO assessment framework

Figure 3.3 Birth registration process in Mexico

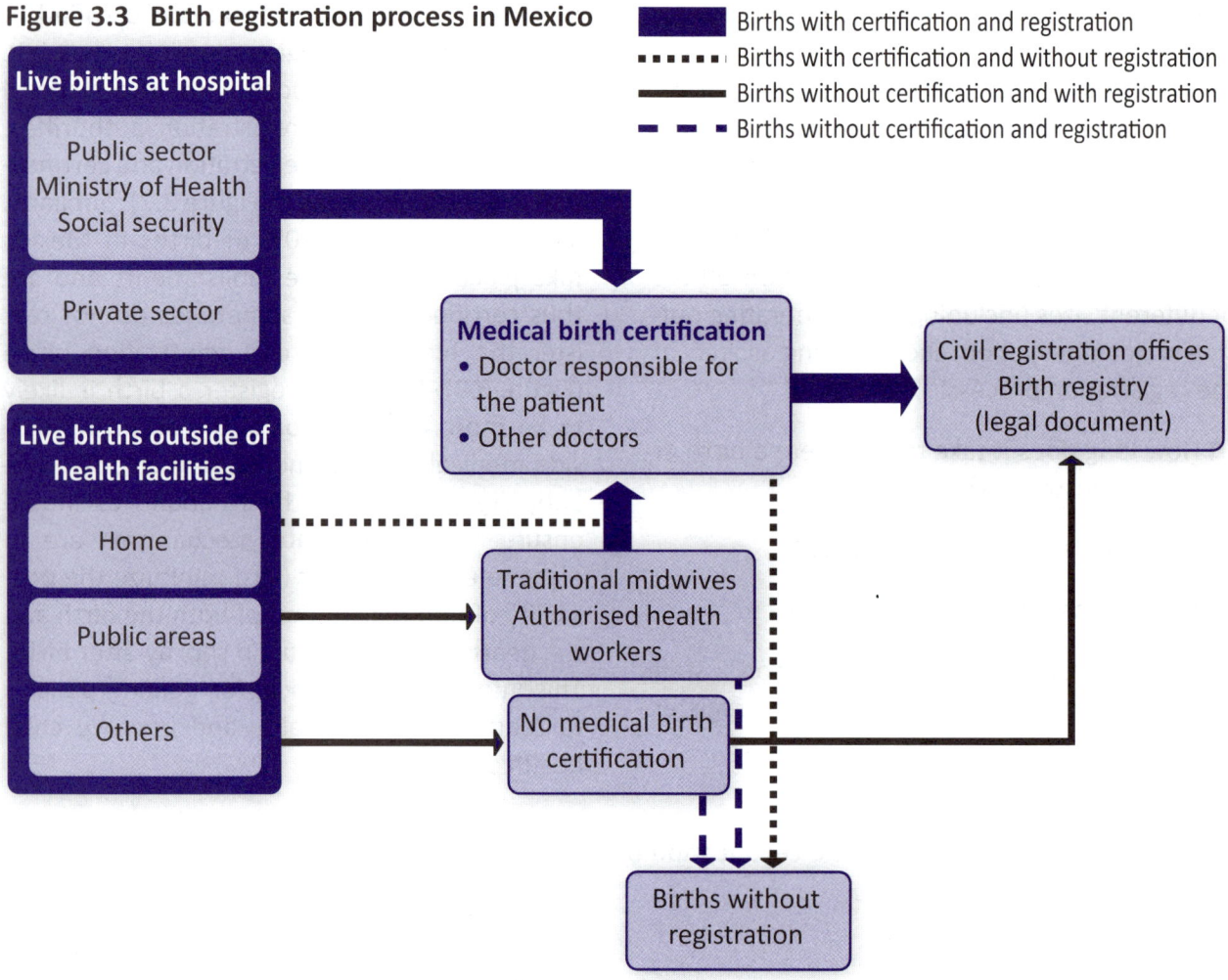

Source: R Lozano, Institute for Health Metrics and Evaluation, University of Washington, personal communication, 2009

The four subcomponents of component B can be assessed by three different subgroups if desired (see Box 2.2). Some questions may need to be reformulated and adapted to suit specific country situations. For example, the questions needed to identify common obstacles to achieving universal registration are likely to differ, depending on the cultural context.

The WHO assessment framework

Subcomponent B1: Organization and functioning of civil registration and vital statistics systems

Supporting material to be prepared in advance:
- Flowchart(s) showing the administrative structures of the civil registration(s) and vital statistics systems, how data flows between them and how they interact.
- Flowchart(s) of the death and birth-registration processes in and outside of hospitals, and for deaths that are handled by the police, coroners or special medical examiners (see Figures 3.2 and 3.3 for examples from Mexico of death and birth registration processes).

Local adaptation of the wording and contents of some questions may be necessary to make them more relevant for assessing the system. This is particularly important in countries where vital statistics are not collected by the civil registration system but by a parallel system.

The many steps between when vital events occur and when they are registered and consolidated into national statistics require good coordination between the different components of the system. The purpose of the review is to discuss any organizational or administrative limitations that may affect the functioning of the system. It is important to focus on the weaker parts or bottlenecks that may decrease the timeliness or quality of the vital statistics.

- **B1.1** What are the organizational and administrative arrangements of the civil registration and vital statistics systems (reviewed using the prepared diagrams)?
- **B1.2** What have been the main changes in the functioning of the systems over the last 10 years?
- **B1.3** How have these changes affected functioning of the system or systems?
- **B1.4** What areas need improvement?

Most countries have separate agencies responsible for the collection of information on vital events (e.g. civil registration) and the production of vital statistics (e.g. a national statistical office or ministry of health). Many countries have formal communication mechanisms between these agencies to ensure smooth coordination and cooperation. Some countries also have broader cooperation committees that meet regularly and include representatives from the health department, hospitals, coroners, police, funeral agencies and religious authorities. Such meetings are particularly important when there is a need to change procedures.

- **B1.5** What are the current communication mechanisms between the civil registration authority and others involved in the collection and production of vital statistics?

Unclear or overlapping responsibilities between agencies can be a major impediment to the smooth functioning of the system and often lead to waste of resources. For instance, is it clear who is responsible for transferring records from one unit to another, or for verifying the data? If someone is absent from work, are there procedures in place to ensure that the person's duties are carried out in a timely fashion?

- **B1.6** Are there any areas where the responsibilities for specific functions overlap or are unclear?
- **B1.7** Are national, state or provincial and local responsibilities clearly defined?
- **B1.8** Are there any areas where bottlenecks regularly occur?

The flowcharts prepared (including those showing detailed birth and death registration practices) should form the basis of discussion. All the steps in the different registration processes (e.g. covering events in and outside hospital) should be included, with a focus on trying to pinpoint where in the process there are leakages that lead to events not being registered. For example, in some countries, the rules may discourage registration of abandoned children or children of under-aged or unmarried mothers.

- **B1.9** Review in detail the country's practices for birth and death registration. Which types of births and deaths are likely to escape the civil registration system?
- **B1.10** Are these types of births and deaths also missed by the vital statistics system?
- **B1.11** Are there some vital events that cannot be registered through the normal system?

Improving the quality and use of birth, death and cause-of-death information

The WHO assessment framework

Subcomponent B1: Organization and functioning of civil registration and vital statistics systems (cont.)

All subnational entities should collect information in a standard format; this will allow comparable national figures to be compiled. This generally requires that a specific national entity be given the task of setting standards and coordinating data collection. In countries where there are separate data collection systems at the state or provincial levels, coordination will be needed.

- **B1.12** Are the same data on births and deaths collected across the country and at every level of the system (including state or provincial, national and local levels)?
- **B1.13** Is there an entity responsible for national vital statistics standards and coordination?

The civil registration system focuses on the birth or death event itself. However, for public health purposes, information on the circumstances of birth and the cause of death are crucial. Cause-of-death information is often collected on a separate form, and sent to the ministry of health as the main user of the data. Medical details related to births are also extremely valuable for identifying subpopulations of children or mothers at risk. Details of particular public health relevance include birth weight, prematurity, birth deformity, birth order (for multiple births), method of delivery and complications.

- **B1.14** Is cause of death included on the death registration form?
- **B1.15** If not, is information about the cause of death collected at the same time as the death is registered but using a different form? Also discuss what happens with coronial cases and deaths from suspected non-natural causes.
- **B1.16** Who decides what details to collect on births and on causes of death?
- **B1.17** How is medical information on births and deaths exchanged among the different government agencies involved?
- **B1.18** Is this process currently working well or does it need improvement?

In many countries the establishment of a "population register" has been a natural extension of the computerization of civil registration and a desire to streamline government agencies and reduce duplication. The population register is derived from the data collected by the civil registration system, and integrates all information on individuals into one record per person, identifiable by a personal identification number (PIN).[4]

- **B1.19** Is there a national population register?
- **B1.20** If so, how does information flow between the national population register and the civil registration system, and which government agency is responsible for maintaining the national population register?
- **B1.21** Is each individual assigned a PIN at birth registration or at the time of receiving identity papers, and is this PIN used throughout the government's administrative databases?
- **B1.22** If a PIN is not given, how are records from various data systems linked, and how is the population register updated?

Computerization of civil registration and vital statistics records cannot by itself improve the quality of the data contained in civil registration records, but it does have a number of advantages. For example, computerization helps to promote timeliness of different processes, including data production and management; it also facilitates the verification, validation and sharing of vital statistics data. If there are plans to expand the computerization of the data system in the near future, it is important to discuss the effect that further computerization is likely to have on the quality and timeliness of the statistics produced.

- **B1.23** Are computers used at any stage of the birth and death registration process?
- **B1.24** Are computers used for any or all of:
  - data compilation?
  - data transmission?
  - data validation?
  - data storage?
- **B1.25** Are there any plans for further computerization in the near future.
- **B1.26** If so, what are the priorities?

---

[4] As a result of computerization, many countries have established national databases for issuing identity papers, which may use personal identifiers. However, most of these databases contain only the adult population and are not connected to the civil registration. They are established for national security, and are not the same as a population register.

Subcomponent B1: Organization and functioning of civil registration and vital statistics systems (cont.)

Systems for checking data for errors or inconsistencies should be in place at all levels of the vital statistics system, beginning at the data collection point. Ideally, a set of standard data checking procedures should be determined centrally and distributed for use at every data collection office. These procedures should include checks on the logic and completeness of the raw data, as well as checks on the arithmetic and logic of the vital statistics once they are compiled.

- **B1.27** What procedures for checking the completeness and consistency of information collected at points of registration are currently being carried out at the points of registration?
- **B1.28** What procedures for checking completeness and consistency of information are carried out at central and other levels?

There should be no large fluctuations from year to year in the numbers of births and deaths registered, as well as causes of death, including deaths without specified causes. If there are large fluctuations, the causes should be investigated, including querying the people who collected the data.

- **B1.29** Are monthly or quarterly registration data routinely checked to ensure that they are comparable with previous years?
- **B1.30** At the central level, are the expected numbers of births and deaths that should occur each year routinely estimated for each registration area, and compared to the actual numbers of registered events?

The WHO assessment framework

Although relatively few questions are suggested for subcomponent B2, the task could involve reviewing a large number of forms. Local adaptation of wording and contents of the questions should be considered before beginning the review.

Subcomponent B2: Review of forms used for birth and death registration

Supporting material to be prepared in advance:
- all forms related to the registration and certification of births and deaths;
- a copy of Box 3.2 (see below), showing a list of topics that the UN recommends be included in birth and death registration.

B2.1 Which of the UN-recommended items are collected on birth and death registration forms? Use Box 3.2 and tick off all items collected.

B2.2 Which of the UN-recommended items that are not collected on the birth and death registration forms would be useful?

B2.3 What additional items are collected on the birth and death registration forms? List and discuss these items.

As increasing numbers of births take place with medical assistance, it is recommended that the birth form include an attachment for collecting medical details about the birth, the baby and the mother. This information is important for improving maternal and child health care, because birth records can be used to identify high-risk infants and mothers for subsequent follow-up. Data other than birth weight might include prematurity, birth order (for multiple births), method of delivery, complications during delivery, stillbirth and date of the mother's most recent delivery.

B2.4 Are any medical details collected (either on the birth registration form or a separate form) regarding the health of the child or the birth process?

The quality of the information obtained is affected by the clarity of the question, the layout of the form (which should be uncluttered and leave sufficient space for adding comments), and the amount of information requested. Errors are also likely to be introduced each time information is transcribed from one form to another.

B2.5 Review all the forms used for registering and certifying births and deaths and answer the following questions for each set of forms:
- Is all the information collected used?
- How long does it take, on average, to fill out each set of forms?
- Is the layout of the forms user-friendly? Explain why or why not.
- Is the form available in each of the main national languages?
- Which items come from the "declarant" and which are transcribed from other documents; for example, is the cause of death transcribed from the death certification form?

The WHO assessment framework

Box 3.2 Recommended list of high-priority characteristics to include in birth and death registration information

The UN recommends that the data collected during registration of a birth or death should include the specific characteristics of the event, of the parents (if a birth) or of the deceased person (if a death). The characteristics listed below have been selected because they are potentially useful for supporting national policy and programme development, and for building and maintaining regional and global comparability.

Although the list shows high-priority characteristics (which ideally should constitute an immediate goal), countries may wish to begin with a shorter list. For example, the long list of parental characteristics may be irrelevant to some countries, or too burdensome. Further, some of this information can be derived from other information and does not need to be asked again. Countries are encouraged to identify their own priorities from the list provided below. However, each country will need to include a registration serial number, the place of registration (or the code of the registration office) and the names of those people directly involved with the event (*1*).

Live births

Characteristics of the event:
- Date of occurrence
- Date of registration
- Place of occurrence
- Place of registration
- Locality of occurrence (derived)
- Urban or rural occurrence (derived)
- Type of birth (i.e. single, twin, triplet, etc.)

Characteristics of the child:
- Sex
- Birth weight

Characteristics of the parents:
- Date of birth and age (derived) of both parents
- Marital status of both parents
- Educational attainment of both parents
- Place of usual residence of both parents
- Locality of residence (derived)
- Urban or rural residence (derived)
- Children born alive to mother during her entire life (to date)
- Children born to mother and who are still living
- Fetal deaths to mother
- Date of last previous live birth
- Date of marriage and duration (derived)

Deaths

Characteristics of the event:
- Date of occurrence
- Date of registration
- Place of occurrence
- Place of registration
- Locality of occurrence (derived)
- Urban or rural occurrence (derived)
- Cause(s) of death
- Certifier and type of certification (derived)

Characteristics of the deceased:
- Date of birth and age (derived)
- Sex
- Marital status
- Place of usual residence (for deaths, less than one year residence of mother)
- Locality of residence (derived)
- Urban or rural residence (derived)

Improving the quality and use of birth, death and cause-of-death information

The WHO assessment framework

> **Box 3.3 Access to civil registration and completeness of vital registration**
>
> As a country develops its civil registration system, it is important to regularly monitor progress. One way to do this is to measure the access that people have to civil registration and the completeness of the registration data, although doing so can be quite complex. For example, access is a complex concept that covers a range of issues, including availability of registration points, distance, affordability, and cultural and social acceptability. This box describes two measures, one of access and one of completeness of registration.
>
> **Access**
>
> Access, as measured by availability, can be calculated by dividing the number of people living in census enumeration districts that have at least one civil registration office or other facility to register births or deaths (numerator in the equation below) by the total national population (denominator) for the same year, and then multiplying by 100 to give a percentage figure.
>
> Thus, access level (in %) can be calculated as $X = C/P \times 100$
>
> | | |
> |---|---|
> | X | Access level in % |
> | C | Size of population in districts with registration points |
> | P | Total population of the country |
>
> **Completeness**
>
> Completeness is a measure of the extent to which the births and deaths that occur in a country in a given year are registered by the civil registration system. Several demographic techniques have been developed to assess and adjust information on births and deaths that come from civil registration. Some methods compare data from independent sources (direct "capture–recapture" approaches) whereas others are indirect analytic methods, based on assumptions about the population age distribution. There are various indirect demographic techniques for estimating the completeness of death registration; for example, the Bennett–Horiuchi, Chanrasekaran–Deming and Brass Growth Balance methods (*1*). These methods are not described in detail here, but are often used by a national statistics office or academic institution to estimate registration completeness.
>
> If such methods have not been applied, a more basic approach is to estimate completeness by dividing the *actual* number of registered births (or deaths) in the country by the total *estimated* number of births (or deaths) in the country for the same period and multiplying by 100 to give a percentage. A simple way to measure completeness in this way is to use an independent estimate of the total number of births (or deaths) in the country. If no reliable national estimate is available, then an international one can be used. For example, each year the UN estimates birth and death rates in its Member States using various sources and demographic estimation techniques (*19*). The reliability of such calculations of registration completeness clearly depends on the reliability of the independent estimates of crude birth rate and crude death rate.
>
> Completeness of birth registration can be calculated as: $YB = (RB/CBR \times P) \times 100$
>
> | | |
> |---|---|
> | YB | Estimated birth registration completeness (%) |
> | RB | Actual number of registered births |
> | CBR | Crude birth rates as estimated by the UN (per 1000) |
> | P | Total population size (in '000s) |
>
> Completeness of death registration can be calculated as: $YD = (RD/CDR \times P) \times 100$
>
> | | |
> |---|---|
> | YD | Estimated death registration completeness (%) |
> | RD | Actual number of registered deaths |
> | CDR | Crude death rates as estimated by the UN (per 1000) |
> | P | Total population size (in '000s) |
>
> **Example**
>
> The UN estimates that the CDR for country A in 2005 was 5.4 per 1000 population. The population of country A in that year was reported as 69,421,000.
>
> If the civil registration system registered 280,510 deaths in 2005, the completeness of death registration in country A would be estimated as follows:
>
> $YD = (280,510/5.4 \times 69,421) = 280,510/374,873 = 74.8\%$

The WHO assessment framework

Subcomponent B3: Coverage and completeness of registration

Supporting material to be prepared in advance:
- calculations of population access to the civil registration system (Box 3.3);
- calculations of the completeness of civil registration data (Box 3.3).

The completeness of registration is closely related to the extent that people have access to registration points. Hence, as the access proportion increases, it is likely that registration completeness will also increase. To calculate the access of the population to vital statistics registration services, countries will need to use census data. Change in access can be calculated from the previous two or three censuses (Box 3.3 shows an example of how to calculate access).

- **B3.1** What proportion of the population has access to civil registration in the area where they live?
- **B3.2** Has access over time:
  - improved? If so, why?
  - remained stable? If so, why?
  - decreased? If so, why?
- **B3.3** If access has improved, what has led to the improvements?

The utility of a vital statistics system depends on the extent to which all events are registered. If the country has not recently evaluated the completeness of the vital statistics data, this should be done using the simple method shown in Box 3.3. If a more complete evaluation was carried out recently (e.g. completeness by age groups using capture–recapture methods), the results from this evaluation should be used.

An analysis of trends in the number of births and deaths that are registered can provide important insights into the status of vital registration efforts in the country. Trends should also be analysed at the subnational level as this can highlight differences in registration coverage in different parts of the country.

- **B3.4** How complete are the birth registration data (i.e. what is the percent completeness level)? Please indicate what method you used to estimate completeness.
- **B3.5** How complete are the death registration data (i.e. what is the percent completeness level)?
- **B3.6** Has completeness over the last decade been:
  - improving? If so, why?
  - stable? If so, why?
  - decreasing? If so, why?

Underregistration cannot be assumed to be the same throughout a country. Births and deaths are less likely to be registered in rural areas and in certain population groups. Also, in some settings, deaths among females are less likely to be registered than deaths among males. It is useful to list any subpopulations that may be being missed by the vital statistics system; for example, people living in remote rural areas, indigenous peoples, nomadic populations and specific age groups, especially neonates.

Some countries have carried out registration campaigns, set up mobile registration, or instituted informal reporting from primary health-care workers to increase the completeness of registration.

- **B3.7** What subpopulations are most likely to be undercounted in vital registration? (Note: undercounting may be different for births and deaths.)
- **B3.8** If only part of the country is covered (e.g. urban areas), have alternative ways of obtaining vital statistics for non-covered populations been considered or implemented; for example, a "sample registration system" (SRS) or a demographic surveillance system (DSS)?
- **B3.9** What has been done in the last 10 years to increase:
  - birth registration?
  - death registration?

Improving the quality and use of birth, death and cause-of-death information

The WHO assessment framework

Subcomponent B3: Coverage and completeness of registration (cont.)

Late registration only becomes a problem where year of occurrence and registration differ. Nonetheless, the extent of late registration should be tracked and monitored to ensure that it is decreasing and not increasing.

B3.10 Is late registration tracked and monitored over time and at the subnational level?

B3.11 Is late registration more common in some areas than others?

Births and deaths that take place in health facilities are more likely to be reported. Hence, as the proportion of these events increases, so should the completeness of registration. Countries that have civil registrars located in hospitals and that have introduced a midwifery reporting system have made substantial improvements in the registration of births and deaths. More generally, matching reported events from hospitals and health facilities with registered vital events provides an estimate of the extent of non-registration.

B3.12 What proportion of registered births take place in health facilities?

B3.13 What proportion of registered deaths take place in health facilities?

B3.14 What proportion of hospitals or other health facilities have registration officers on the premises?

B3.15 Do midwives or other health personnel attending home births also report these births? If so, to whom?

B3.16 Are reported births from such sources routinely compared with registered births?

The reporting of births and deaths occurring in private institutions may be poor if not compulsory and specified by law.

B3.17 What proportion of births take place in nongovernmental health facilities?

B3.18 What proportion of deaths take place in nongovernmental health facilities?

It is generally recommended that there should be no charge for initial registration of births and deaths and issuing of original certificates. A fee is commonly charged for issue of subsequent copies of birth and death certificates.

B3.19 Does registration involve any financial costs to the family or informant:
- **for births?**
- **for deaths?**

Some countries have maternity or child allowances that the mother can access, provided she can produce a birth certificate. Also, a death certificate is usually needed to claim insurance, pension benefits and inheritance. Discuss how access to other benefits might potentially increase registration completeness.

An increasing number of countries have introduced obligatory identity cards for the adult population, and a birth certificate is often needed to prove identity to get the card. This has undoubtedly increased awareness among the population of the utility of registering birth.

B3.20 What social services or benefits are linked to birth registration?

B3.21 What social services, insurance benefits or inheritance transfers are linked to death registration?

B3.22 If the country uses identity cards, how does that system affect vital events registration?

Subcomponent B3: Coverage and completeness of registration (cont.)

It is useful to list the main obstacles and deterrents that may discourage people from registering births and death, and to then discuss each of these and propose how each of these may be overcome or reduced.

B3.23 What are the main obstacles to improving civil registration? For example:
- lack of registrars or places to register;
- lack of access to health facilities;
- lack of knowledge about the need to register births and deaths;
- social stigma of illegitimate children;
- cultural barriers;
- financial barriers;
- illiteracy;
- shortage of physicians and midwives;
- other obstacles (please specify).

It is also useful to discuss any improvements that resulted from the most recent campaign to increase public awareness of the utility of civil registration, and to outline further improvements that could be made.

B3.24 When did the country last have a campaign to increase public awareness of the need to register vital events?

B3.25 Were the results evaluated?

B3.26 Is there a committee that regularly monitors and evaluates civil registration completeness?

The WHO assessment framework

Subcomponent B4: Data storage and transmission

Supporting material to be prepared in advance:

- Separate flowcharts of how data on birth and death registration are transmitted from the local level to higher levels and the central storage facility (include how often the data are transmitted and how the data are transmitted).

- A separate flowchart of how data from civil registration (and other sources recording vital events) are transmitted to the unit preparing vital statistics. (Note: the extent to which the civil registration and vital statistics systems are integrated or function as separate systems varies among countries and will determine whether many of the questions need to be duplicated to cover all the flows in both systems.)

The UN has produced a series of handbooks to guide countries on civil registration; two of these handbooks are particularly relevant for data management and maintenance of civil registration records (20, 25).

- **B4.1** Do local registration offices record and store the collected information on births and deaths by:
  - registry books?
  - electronic files?
  - other (please specify)?
- **B4.2** Are birth and death records filed by:
  - date of registration?
  - name?
  - a numbering system or other numerical index?
  - other (please specify)?

There are different ways of storing and archiving records. A major requirement of any system is to ensure that registrars can retrieve individual records to make copies and issue certificates. Hence, a proper filing and archiving system is crucial. Long-term storage and preservation is usually best done at a national level and is easier to do with electronic records. However, where registration records are not computerized, copies also need to be stored at the local level so that local authorities and individuals have ready access. When records are computerized, daily backup of electronic files is recommended, to ensure that records are not lost if equipment fails.

- **B4.3** What method of record backup is used and how frequently is this done?
- **B4.4** How are birth and death records archived?
- **B4.5** Have records ever been lost or destroyed?
- **B4.6** How can the loss or destruction of records be avoided in the future?
- **B4.7** Can individual birth or death records easily be retrieved if needed?

Because birth records in many countries are used for establishing identity cards and legal documents, they are more often subject to fraud. Vital records should not be treated as public documents, and certificates should only be issued to those with a legitimate right to ask for them. To avoid abuse, some countries have instituted a surveillance programme that requests information on the birth record that only the registrant would normally know; for example, maiden name of mother. Many countries also mark the birth records with the word "deceased" when the person dies.

- **B4.8** Have there been instances of fraudulent or multiple registrations?
- **B4.9** What precautions are built into the system to avoid fraudulent or multiple registrations?

Depending on the type of system and infrastructure available, there are many possible ways to consolidate and transfer data from the birth and death registration forms to create vital statistics. However, wherever data consolidation is performed – be it manually, mechanically or electronically – errors can occur; therefore, routine checking of data outputs is recommended.

- **B4.10** Using the flowcharts of data transmission prepared for birth and death records, explain where and how data are being consolidated before transmission.

Subcomponent B4: Data storage and transmission (cont.)

Reporting all vital events according to a fixed time schedule is a cornerstone of successful civil registration and vital statistics systems. Routine follow-up should be made to civil registration offices if the offices do not report on time. Every delay in reporting affects the timeliness of the national data and decreases the potential effectiveness of any query about the data in cases where information is missing or judged to be incorrect.

- **B4.11** Reflecting on the data-flowchart prepared, is there a fixed schedule for transferring data in a timely manner?
- **B4.12** Is this schedule strictly adhered to?
- **B4.13** Is this schedule routinely monitored by those receiving the data?
- **B4.14** Are there procedures in place to deal with late or non-reporting from local civil registration offices?
- **B4.15** If there are procedures in place, what are they?

People may be discouraged from registering births and deaths if the public perception is that the confidentiality of information reported on birth and death registration forms is not guaranteed. Also, doctors may not feel comfortable reporting accurate cause-of-death information if the record is not considered confidential.

- **B4.16** Is the information on the birth and death registration forms kept confidential?
- **B4.17** How is confidentiality maintained?
- **B4.18** Who can access the data and for what purposes?

Errors in the data can happen both at the time of registering the event and when data are consolidated, transcribed and transferred. Hence, it is recommended that the office receiving the statistics routinely checks the data. This is much easier if the data are computerized. In cases where there are queries with the transferred data, rapid feedback to local registration offices is essential, so allow the data to be corrected. This also encourages local offices to improve data quality.

- **B4.19** What checks are made on individual birth and death records to ensure that they are accurate and complete when transferred?
- **B4.20** Are local registration offices routinely contacted for clarification about the statistics by the regional or central level?
- **B4.21** If so, how frequently is clarification sought?

Local offices should be able to provide the data they collect to local authorities for local planning; they should also know how the data compare with the national situation. Thus, the central office producing the country's vital statistics must keep the local offices informed about how their areas are performing in terms of birth and death rates, compared to the national context.

- **B4.22** Is there two-way communication and data transfer between central and peripheral offices?
- **B4.23** Do regional registration authorities routinely receive reports on how the characteristics of their populations compare with the national average?

3.5 Component C – Death certification and cause of death

This section covers component C – *Death certification and cause of death* – within which are the following subcomponents:

- C1 – ICD-compliant practices for death certification (*24*);
- C2 – Hospital death certification;
- C3 – Deaths occurring outside hospital;
- C4 – Practices affecting the quality of cause-of-death data.

In properly functioning civil registration and vital statistics systems, all births and deaths in the population are recorded. With regard to cause-of-death statistics, the gold standard (i.e. the ideal) is complete civil registration, where

The WHO assessment framework

each death has the underlying cause assigned by a medically qualified doctor (for best practice in death certification, see Centers for Disease Control and Prevention, 2007 (*26*)) and coded by someone trained in the ICD rules and principles (*27*). The principle of using the "underlying cause of death" for tabulating cause of death statistics can be applied uniformly by using the *International form of medical certificate of cause of death*, which is shown in Box 3.4. This form was designed for making it easier to select the underlying cause of death when two or more causes are recorded on the death certificate.

Box 3.4   International form of medical certificate of cause of death

Death certificates are the main source of mortality data. A properly completed certificate of death shows clearly why and how the death occurred; it also contains key personal characteristics of the deceased person. The parts of this certificate that give information on cause of death (Parts I and II), and a section to record the time interval between the onset of each condition and the date of death, are shown below.

In completing the certificate, the certifier should report any disease, abnormality, injury or external cause that is believed to have contributed to the death. Modes of death (e.g. respiratory failure and heart failure) should not be considered as causes of death.

INTERNATIONAL FORM OF MEDICAL CERTIFICATE OF CAUSE OF DEATH

	Cause of death	Approximate interval between onset and death
I Disease or condition directly leading to death*	(a)	....
	due to (or as a consequence of)	
Antecedent causes Morbid conditions, if any, giving rise to the above cause, stating the underlying condition last	(b)	....
	due to (or as a consequence of)	
	(c)	....
	due to (or as a consequence of)	
	(d)	....
II Other significant conditions contributing to the death, but not related to the disease or condition causing it	....	....

*This does not mean the mode of dying, e.g. heart failure, respiratory failure. It means the disease, injury, or complication that caused death.

Source: WHO (2007) (*28*)

The four subcomponents of component C investigate the extent to which the current system correctly records the cause of death, as well as national practices that might affect the quality of the reporting. Given the specific knowledge required to answer some of the questions, the subgroup must include physicians with death certification experience.

Only about 70 WHO member countries produce cause-of-death data of acceptable quality from their civil registration and vital statistics systems (*12*). In the other 50 or so countries that produce some cause-of-death data, the quality of the information is poor because of poor certification and coding practices. Most deaths in these countries that occur outside hospitals are not medically certified, and a high proportion of these deaths are assigned to non-specific or "ill-defined causes" (e.g. old age, fever, stopped breathing, etc). These vague diagnoses are of no use for public health purposes.

Studies examining the causes of poor certification in developing countries are rare, but the limited information that exists suggests that inaccuracies in the data are mostly derived from characteristics of the certifier (e.g. no training), the certificate (e.g. not aligned with ICD practice), the deceased person (e.g. older age groups) and the cause of death (e.g. sudden death) (29). Further, in many countries the value of routine data collections for public health progress and population health is not appreciated; hence, there are not sufficient regulations and procedures to ensure that medical certification and coding of cause of death are done correctly.

The collaboration and compliance of health practitioners and hospitals is crucial for the proper attribution of cause of death. Collaboration and compliance are difficult to achieve in countries with weak legal frameworks or poor governance. In cases of sudden death, it is also necessary to have someone who is medically trained to assess whether a death can be considered as natural (due to disease) or due to some external cause (accident, suicide or homicide). In many countries, deaths due to external causes are referred to a coroner or special medical examiner, or are handled by the police, who are then responsible for assigning the cause of death.

When a death occurs in a medical establishment or other setting where a doctor is present to certify the cause of death, the process is initiated by the doctor completing a death certificate. The family of the deceased can then use the certificate to register the death and obtain a burial permit. In many developed countries, the doctor sends a copy of the certificate to the undertaker responsible for disposing of the body. It is the undertaker who must register the death with the civil registration authority, to get permission to transport and dispose of the body.

In countries where there is a shortage of medical doctors in rural areas, it is often the village leader who provides a lay opinion about the cause of death. This is not best practice and these data should never be combined with cause-of-death data that are medically certi-

fied. While the event of death can usually be recognized by a layperson, the cause of death has to be correctly diagnosed by a qualified medical doctor.

Even where medical certification of the cause of death is common practice, it does not necessarily mean that the correct cause of death is written on the death certificate in the correct way. Most doctors certify death infrequently, and their medical school training may have been forgotten or be out of date. Lack of diagnostic facilities, human error, inexperience and lack of awareness of the importance of cause-of-death data all contribute to poor diagnostic accuracy. Further, there may be financial or social consequences for the family that deter the doctor from reporting the true cause of death. Examples include life-insurance schemes that reimburse medical expenses for certain health conditions only, or the social stigma associated with HIV/AIDS and drug overdose.

Deaths from external causes are frequently underreported. Although accidents and violence typically account for about 10% of all deaths (and an even higher percentage in some countries), they are often systematically undercounted by civil registration systems (30). Among the most important reasons for this underreporting is the legal requirement that deaths due to accidents and violence be investigated by the police or a coroner (Box 3.5). In such cases, the cause of death may be initially registered as not defined or unknown, pending the outcome of the investigation. It is common for there to be significant delays in finalizing the data, and the true cause of death may never be corrected in the vital statistics system. Accidental deaths may also be missed if the ICD rules are not correctly applied, and the cause of death is attributed to the immediate condition that led to death (e.g. pneumonia), instead of to the underlying injury that precipitated the sequence of morbid conditions that led to death. These issues are examined further in the questions for this component.

The WHO assessment framework

> **Box 3.5 Special enquiry systems**
>
> Unnatural deaths include deaths caused by accidents, suicides and homicides; deaths with unknown causes; deaths in which the deceased person did not see a doctor in the preceding three months; and certain special cases (e.g. deaths occurring in prison or during anaesthesia). In many countries, all unnatural deaths are referred to special enquiry, often by a coroner or special medical examiner who carries out an investigation into the circumstances surrounding the death. The types of deaths subject to a special enquiry are laid down in a coroners Act or other regulations.
>
> In some countries, coroners are usually magistrates, employed by the department of justice. Police officers assist coroners or special examiners with their enquiries into the cause of death. A postmortem examination is often ordered to establish the medical cause of death. A postmortem is a detailed internal and external examination of the body by a pathologist or government medical officer. During a postmortem, all parts of the body are inspected thoroughly to determine the presence, nature and extent of any disease or injury. In most cases, laboratory tests are also needed. Tests can include microscopic examination of tissue samples from the major organs, and may include chemical analysis for drugs, alcohol or poisons.

A systematic examination and discussion of the questions and issues raised in the four subcomponents (C1–C4) will generate insights into medical certification practices and will help to determine what needs to be changed to improve the quality and utility of cause-of-death statistics. Important public health decisions are taken based on cause-of-death data, and it is essential that the information provided by doctors on death certificates is accurate and reliable.

> **Subcomponent C1: ICD-compliant practices for death certification**
>
> **Supporting material to be prepared in advance:**
> - Copy of the international form of medical certificate of cause of death (Box 3.4).
> - Copies of all forms used to collect death and cause-of-death information (e.g. forms for deaths in and outside hospitals; and forms used by police, coroners, civil registries, etc.).
> - A diagram that explains how unnatural deaths from accidents, suicides and homicides are dealt with and shows how these data are fed into the cause-of-death database.
>
> A medically certified cause of death, in which a physician has completed the death certificate and given a judgement on the cause of death, is the gold standard for generating cause-of-death information. As a general rule, the higher the proportion of deaths that are medically certified, the more reliable the resulting cause-of-death statistics. The percentage of registered deaths that are medically certified can be calculated as the number of deaths registered with a medically certified cause of death, divided by total registered deaths multiplied by 100.
>
> **C1.1 How many registered deaths (as a percentage) have a medically certified cause of death?**
>
> Lay-reported causes are causes of death assigned by anyone other than a medical doctor, such as a village or group leader, police officer or registrar. These cases should always be reported separately in cause-of-death tabulations. This is important because the value of the information is different. Medically certified causes allow for more-detailed classification and analysis.
>
> **C1.2 In the cause-of-death data, is it possible to separate medically certified deaths and those certified by a layperson?**
>
> **C1.3 Are these data compiled separately in the cause of death statistics for the country?**

The WHO assessment framework

Subcomponent C1: ICD-compliant practices for death certification (cont.)

Volume 2 of the ICD provides global guidelines and standards for mortality certification as well as the rules and procedures for selecting the underlying cause of death (*28*). It also explains why the underlying cause of death, rather than the immediate cause, should be used for tabulation of the cause of death. The international form of medical certificate of cause of death (Box 3.4) was designed so that these principles could be applied uniformly in all settings and the resulting cause-of-death statistics could be comparable across time and place.

- **C1.4** Are ICD-compliant practices used for death certification in the country?
- **C1.5** Is the standard international form of medical certificate of cause of death (Box 3.4) used for:
  - all deaths?
  - only deaths occurring in hospitals not for those taken place outside hospitals?
  - only deaths occurring in some specific hospitals, such as university or regional hospitals?
  - other deaths (please specify)?

Introduction of the *International form of medical certificate of cause of death* will need to be coordinated through a wide-ranging information campaign directed at medical practitioners and health statisticians, to ensure that the concepts on the certificate, and the reasons for collecting the data, are well understood.

- **C1.6** If the country does not use the standard *International form of medical certificate of cause of death*, how could it be introduced (specify steps)? What potential actions (e.g. sensitization of medical establishment) would be required?

Understanding what is meant by the underlying cause of death is essential for correctly certifying deaths and producing statistics that are useful for health planning and disease prevention.

- **C1.7** Do doctors know how to correctly complete the death certificate, including the causal sequence and the underlying cause?
  - Yes, generally.
  - Yes, always.
  - No, they do not.

Some countries have prepared written materials (booklets and brochures) that provide a low-cost way to help doctors to correctly fill in the death certificate.

- **C1.8** Is there a booklet, brochure or other guideline for doctors explaining how to certify the cause of death and complete the international form properly?
- **C1.9** If such material is not available, what would be involved in preparing it and how could it be distributed?

With the exception of deaths due to an accident or injury, where only one cause is usually present, most deaths result from a sequence of events involving more than one disease or condition. Even though the underlying cause of death is the only cause coded, the certifying doctor must mention all the main contributing diseases and conditions, to allow the coder to select the correct underlying cause. Including information on the length of time that the deceased person had the specific morbid conditions will also assist with proper certification and coding. The cause of death should not be confused with the "mode of death" (e.g. heart failure, respiratory arrest, etc.). The higher the proportion of death certificates with only one cause listed, or with a mode of death reported, the poorer the quality of death data will usually be. It may be necessary to review a sample of death certificates to explore these issues.

- **C1.10** What proportion of death certificates list only one cause of death? (See Box 3.4 about the need to state not only the disease directly leading to death, but also the underlying conditions without which the person would not have died.)
- **C1.11** What proportion of death certificates report the mode of death instead of the underlying cause of death?
- **C1.12** What proportion of death certificates do not indicate the interval between onset of disease and death?

Improving the quality and use of birth, death and cause-of-death information

The WHO assessment framework

Subcomponent C2: Hospital death certification

The quality of cause-of-death data will depend on the certifier's ability to diagnose diseases, knowledge of the patient's medical history, and ability to enter this information correctly on the death certificate. Certifying the correct cause of death takes experience; interns and junior doctors should only certify deaths when supervised by more experienced physicians.

- C2.1 In hospitals, who completes the death certificate:
  - the attending doctor?
  - another doctor who did not treat the deceased person before death occurred?
  - a nurse?
  - a medical records officer?
  - other (please specify)?

Attributing correct cause of death is difficult in cases when the deceased person was dead-on-arrival (DOA; i.e. was brought to the hospital but died before any medical intervention could take place). As a result, these deaths are often assigned to ill-defined causes. Some hospitals refuse to certify such deaths and refer them to coroners or special medical examiners. To assess data quality, it is important to know how hospitals certify DOA cases, and how common these cases are.

- C2.2 How are cases of DOA certified?
- C2.3 How common are DOA deaths in hospitals? Do they constitute:
  - less than 10% of deaths?
  - 10–20% of deaths?
  - more than 20% of deaths?

In some countries, deaths can be registered at the hospital, either at hospital registration points or because the hospital forwards the completed registration papers to the civil registration office. These approaches are preferable to relying on individuals to go to the civil registration to register. Figure 3.2 illustrates this point, and demonstrates how certified deaths may not always be registered.

- C2.4 Are the vital events that take place in hospitals registered in the country:
  - at civil registration points in hospitals?
  - by the hospital sending forms to the civil registration office?
  - by the individual family registering after the birth or death has occurred?

The WHO assessment framework

Subcomponent C3: Deaths occurring outside hospital

The quality of cause-of-death data when deaths occur at home depends heavily on whether a doctor is the certifier. In some countries, family doctors certify death by writing the cause of death on plain stationery; this is not good practice. To standardize the cause-of-death information, all doctors should use the same form, which should be issued free-of-charge by the office with authority for collecting cause-of-death data.

- **C3.1** Is it mandatory to issue a death certificate with the cause of death indicated for people who die at home?
- **C3.2** If so, are there any quality problems with these certificates and are they ever reviewed?
- **C3.3** Is the same cause-of-death form used for deaths in and outside hospital?
- **C3.4** If a different form is used for deaths outside hospital, what information is recorded about the cause of death?

If cause-of-death forms can be completed by laypeople (such as village officials) or by doctors who may not have attended the deceased person, the reliability of the assigned cause-of-death will be questionable.

- **C3.5** Who prepares the death certificate and certifies the cause of death for people dying outside of hospital:
  - a general practitioner?
  - a coroner or similar?
  - a health official?
  - a civil registrar?
  - other (please specify)?
- **C3.6** If a doctor is needed, is that person required to examine the deceased person before they have died?
- **C3.7** How are deaths certified in cases where the certifying physician is not the person who treated the patient?

Access to the deceased person's medical records will help doctors to more reliably diagnose the underlying cause of death, particularly for persons dying following long-term illness.

- **C3.8** Are hospital medical records usually accessible to general practitioners when one of their patients dies at home?

When medical certification is not possible, "verbal autopsy" (see Box 3.6, below) is a viable way of obtaining information on important causes of death in parts of the country.

- **C3.9** Is verbal autopsy routinely used to obtain the cause of death for any non-medically certified deaths in the country?
- **C3.10** If verbal autopsy procedures are routinely used, do they conform to the WHO standards (*31*)?
- **C3.11** Has the WHO standard procedure been modified in any way to make it more applicable to the country? (If so, please specify the modification.)

Box 3.6 Verbal autopsy

Verbal autopsy is a way of determining the cause of death by asking caregivers, friends or family members about signs and symptoms experienced by the deceased person in the period before death. This is usually done with a standard questionnaire that collects details on signs, symptoms and any medical history or events prior to death.

The cause of death or the sequence of causes that led to death should always be assigned by a doctor, based on this questionnaire and all other available information. Guidelines and diagnostic algorithms are available to assist in evaluating the information and correctly diagnosing the cause of death (*31*).

The purpose of a verbal autopsy is to obtain information on cause of death at the community or population level where vital registration with medical certification is limited or absent.

The WHO assessment framework

Subcomponent C4: Practices affecting the quality of cause-of-death data

Country practices vary as to who has access to cause-of-death information. Sometimes the part of the form containing the cause of death is sent straight to the vital statistics unit at the ministry of health or national statistics office for processing, and details are not kept by the civil registration offices. In other cases, the civil registration system records only broad causes of death, and forwards detailed data on causes of death to the office responsible for vital statistics. Countries also vary in the extent to which cause of death is considered confidential information. In some, it is considered an extension of the doctor–patient relationship and only shared with the closest family and medical authorities; in others, it is freely available.

- **C4.1** To whom, other than the family, is the cause-of-death information for individuals provided (including upon request)?
- **C4.2** What information is provided to the family on the death certificate:
  - all the information on the cause-of-death form?
  - an extract for laypersons about the cause of death?
  - other (please specify)?

In many countries, some causes of death are widely viewed as unacceptable, either because of stigmatization, superstition or the risk of non-payment by insurance companies. Pressure from the family of the deceased may influence the doctor who certifies the death, particularly if that doctor is also the family doctor. While these influences may be difficult to prevent, it is important to understand how they might affect the quality of cause-of-death data.

- **C4.3** Is it likely that many cases with a sensitive or stigmatizing cause of death (e.g. suicide or HIV/AIDS) would be assigned to a more socially acceptable cause of death?

Infant mortality and maternal mortality are widely used indicators for assessing a country's health status and the performance of its health system. Maternal mortality is particularly difficult to measure accurately, because deaths during pregnancy are relatively rare and are often missed or misclassified to other causes. This is particularly likely to happen when the death occurs early in pregnancy (before the fact that the women was pregnant is known), or some time after delivery (when the fact that the women had been pregnant may not be entered in the records). To avoid missing such deaths, the death certificate should include a checkbox prompting the certifying doctor to indicate whether a woman of reproductive age who died was pregnant at the time of death or had recently been pregnant. The Glossary includes definitions of "maternal mortality" and "maternal death".

- **C4.4** Does the death certificate state whether a woman was pregnant, or had recently been pregnant?

In some countries, the death registration system provides a starting point for special reviews of deaths among women of reproductive age, to identify all such deaths that might have been associated with pregnancy but were not classified as such in the death certificate. Reviews of medical records and interviews with care providers and family members are used to build a more complete picture of the circumstances leading to the death, and to permit reclassification of some deaths of reproductive women to maternal causes (*32*).

In many hospital settings, detailed clinical audits of all maternal deaths are conducted to investigate the causes and circumstances surrounding maternal deaths, and to identify possible failings in the availability or quality of care. These audits have been effective in identifying maternal deaths and their causes; they also provide important information to guide national programmes to reduce maternal mortality. Because maternal mortality and perinatal mortality are closely linked, measurement of maternal deaths has also led to strengthened procedures to measure perinatal mortality.

- **C4.5** Are maternal deaths reviewed separately from other deaths?
- **C4.6** Are perinatal deaths monitored using a special form, as recommended by the WHO?

Subcomponent C4: Practices affecting the quality of cause-of-death data (cont.)

If doctors have received little training in how to correctly complete the death certificate, and are not aware of its importance for public health purposes, they will be unable to certify deaths reliably and accurately.[5]

- C4.7 What training and practice do doctors receive in certifying the cause of death:
  - none?
  - one lecture in medical school or at the hospital?
  - an ICD-compliant training course on certification?
  - on-the-job training?
  - other (please specify)?
- C4.8 Would most doctors be aware of the important public health uses of the information they provide on the death certificate?

One way of assessing the quality of death certification is to select a random sample of about 1% of hospital death certificates, and conduct an independent verification of the cause of death using the full set of hospital medical records for the deceased persons. If there are significant differences in the underlying cause of death between the original and the later sources, this indicates the need for retraining of doctors and stricter hospital processes for certifying cause of death. Such evaluations should always be accompanied by an analysis of types of error, so that they can be targeted in the follow-up training.

- C4.9 Has the country evaluated the quality of medical certification?
- C4.10 If yes:
  - When was the evaluation done?
  - How was it done?
  - What did it conclude?
  - What follow-up was undertaken to improve certification practices?

Because there is often more than one condition present at the time of death, doctors need full access to the patient's medical records, as well as technological and other diagnostic aids in order to be able to correctly diagnose the underlying cause of death.

- C4.11 Are hospital medical records generally:
  - complete?
  - reliable?
  - easily accessible to the certifier?
- C4.12 Are other health records, such as from health clinics, general practitioners or family doctors:
  - complete?
  - reliable?
  - easily accessible to the certifier?

Although the ICD provides special instructions on the classification of unnatural deaths, individual countries decide who should be responsible for their certification. Because certification of these deaths is often delayed through judicial investigations (see Box 3.5), they may be missed by the vital statistics system.

The diagram prepared on this topic (see subcomponent C1) should be used for the discussion.

- C4.13 Who certifies whether the cause of death is unnatural (i.e. accident, suicide or homicide)?
- C4.14 If there is a special system for certifying these deaths, please describe how this works and how well it works.

---

[5]See Core curriculum for certifiers of underlying cause of death at http://www.cdc.gov/nchs/injury/injury_matrices.htm

The WHO assessment framework

> **Subcomponent C4: Practices affecting the quality of cause-of-death data (cont.)**
>
> When injury, poisoning or certain other consequences of external causes is the cause of death, the certifier must also describe the circumstances of the incident or accident that led to death. Moreover, the certifier should select this original incident or accident as the underlying cause of death and code it according to Chapter XX of the ICD (V01-Y89). The type of injury or poisoning (Chapter XLX of the ICD Codes S00-T98) may be used as an additional code but should *not* be reported as being the underlying cause. Some countries have a separate box on the death certificate to report on the circumstances surrounding such violent or unnatural deaths.
>
> **C4.15** Are certifying doctors aware of how to report deaths from injuries and external causes according to the ICD rules?

3.6 Component D – ICD mortality coding practices

This section covers component D – ICD mortality coding – within which are the following subcomponents:

- D1 – Mortality coding practices;
- D2 – Mortality coder qualification and training;
- D3 – Quality of mortality coding.

It is not sufficient that the *certification* of cause of death is correctly done according to ICD rules, it is also essential that the *coding* of the cause of death is correct and is compliant with ICD rules and standards.

Most deaths are associated with multiple medical conditions, all of which may have contributed to the death. The international standards provide rules for selecting the cause of death most important or relevant to public health; that is, the underlying cause that gave rise to the chain of other conditions associated with the death. Correctly selecting the underlying cause of death and coding it according to ICD rules and procedures is not a trivial matter; it requires training and skills development. Where the importance of coding mortality data correctly is not understood, information that is needed for development of health policies can be lost.

The coding practices currently in use are best assessed by a subgroup of technically qualified people knowledgeable in national coding practices and the ICD. When delivering their conclusions, the subgroup should make clear that the correct coding of the underlying cause of death depends on the quality of the medical certification. This close relationship has to be carefully explained to the larger stakeholder group so that any deficiencies in the cause-of-death statistics can be discussed as part of the overall cause-of-death certification review. The questions in the three following subcomponents (D1–D3) should help countries to assess how well their procedures for coding causes of death are working, and to identify where weaknesses exist.

The WHO assessment framework

Subcomponent D1: Mortality coding practices

Countries are strongly advised to use the alphanumeric codes of the ICD classification for coding and classifying deaths, and to use the latest version of the ICD, which is currently the 10th revision, 2nd edition (ICD-10) (*28*). If this ICD version is not being used, it is important to discuss the specific steps required to upgrade to ICD-10. Correct application of the ICD will be easier if a version is available in one (or more) of the national languages. It is particularly important to compile a list of locally used medical terms, and include this in the alphabetical index volume (see Volume 3 of ICD-10).

- **D1.1** Is the ICD used for cause-of-death statistics?
- **D1.2** If so, which revision and edition is currently being used?
- **D1.3** Is a national-language version of the ICD used?
- **D1.4** Who is responsible for coordinating the implementation of the ICD?
- **D1.5** Who is responsible for training ICD coders?

The basic ICD classification is a list of three-character categories, each of which can be further divided into up to 10 four-character subcategories. When coding skills and resources are limited, it is useful and sometimes necessary to code to a less detailed summary list of categories. Although summary lists reduce the precision of coding (because each category represents a group of diseases rather than a single disease or injury entity), using these larger aggregates tends to diminish the public health impact of diagnostic and coding errors, and improve comparability. Volume 1 of the ICD-10 contains recommended tabulation lists intended for use in circumstances where the three-character list is too detailed.

- **D1.6** Are the codes selected for cause-of-death reporting chosen from the complete ICD list, or is coding done from a summary tabulation list of the ICD?
- **D1.7** If a summary list is used, which list is it?

In-depth knowledge and understanding of the purpose and structure of the ICD are vital for statisticians, analysts and coders if they are to interpret and code the information on the cause-of-death certificate correctly. Application of the ICD principles and correct use of the selection rules by all coders is crucial to accurately identify the main causes of death in populations and allow international comparisons.

- **D1.8** Are coding and ICD selection rules for underlying cause-of-death data applied?

In some countries, mortality coding is done centrally, often in the ministry of health or national statistical office; in other countries, coding is done in hospitals where the death occurred. Centralized coding of cause of death facilitates the application of common standards and procedures, it is also likely to make error detection and correction easier. In decentralized coding systems used in hospitals, it is easier to access the patient records in case of doubt about the certification, but it is difficult to avoid a certain amount of local interpretation, which could well result in national data inconsistencies.

- **D1.9** Is mortality coding centralized or decentralized?
- **D1.10** If coding is decentralized, what quality measures and procedures are in place to ensure national consistency in the application of ICD coding rules?

To verify and select the correct underlying cause of death, coders should have access to all the information provided on the death certificate. It is not good practice to provide coders only with the cause of death reported by the certifier. Rather, the coder should have access to the original death certificate form, and to all the diseases and injuries reported on the form. This facilitates the selection of the underlying cause of death, and makes it possible to apply the modification tables from the *Automated Classification of Medical Entities* (ACME). It also allows multiple-cause-of-death analysis.

- **D1.11** Is cause-of-death coding done from a copy of the original death certificate or from a transcribed list provided by the civil registration office, or from some other summary document?
- **D1.12** Is all the information on the death certificate coded, or only the presumed underlying cause of death?

The WHO assessment framework

Subcomponent D1: Mortality coding practices (cont.)

In cases where the death certificate does not provide enough information for the coder to select the underlying cause of death, or where the information reported is incorrect, a system for querying doctors for further information is needed.

D1.13 Is there an established mechanism to query the certifier (doctor) in cases where the coder cannot understand or interpret the reported causes of death on the certificate?

D1.14 If so, please describe these procedures and discuss their efficacy.

Subcomponent D2: Mortality coder qualification and training

Compile a list of the ICD training courses that have been offered in the last 3 years. As far as possible, include a summary list of the subject matter taught (see Box 3.7).

In some countries, coding is done by the same physicians who certify the cause of death. More commonly, coding is done by administrative clerks and statisticians who have been specially trained for this task; this is preferable because it fosters the development of a specific cadre of specialized coders who have in-depth knowledge of the ICD rules and procedures.

D2.1 What categories of staff (e.g. physicians, statisticians, and health professionals) are doing mortality coding in the country?

D2.2 What level of education do mortality coders typically have?

All coders should follow a formal training course on correct coding of death certificates. On-the-job training is important, but training courses with standardized curricula ensure consistency of knowledge transfer. It is useful to compare the country's coder training with the sample curriculum shown in Box 3.7. The material on training prepared in advance should be used in the discussion of these questions.

To ensure consistency in levels of skills, training curricula and courses should be standardized nationally. Senior ICD trainers are required for local sustainability of coding skills.

D2.3 Are specific training courses provided for mortality coders or do they learn on-the-job?

D2.4 If coders are specifically trained to code:
- Are there sufficient local ICD trainers to meet the needs?
- Who is responsible for delivering the training?
- What is the length of training and is there a standard curriculum?
- How often is coder training conducted?

To avoid a high turnover of coders, their skills and qualification should be formally recognized, with diplomas issued for the professional titles bestowed as a result of successful training. Career paths are important for retaining trained coders.

D2.5 Is there a high turnover among coders?

D2.6 Are coders recognized within staffing structures as a separate cadre, and are coding qualifications recognized separately to other administrative officers?

The WHO Collaborating Centres Network for the Family of International Classifications[6] ("WHO-FIC") regularly offers training courses in ICD coding. Additional training in medical terminology and medical science can improve the skills of coders. Training is also required for coders when applying new versions of the ICD, or when the local adaptation of the ICD has been changed.

D2.7 Are there local senior trainers who have been trained at WHO-FIC supported training courses?

D2.8 Do coders have opportunities for ongoing education?

---

[6] http://www.who.int/classifications/network/en/

The WHO assessment framework

Box 3.7 Summarized training curriculum for coders

As a result of collaboration between WHO-FIC and the International Federation of Health Records Organizations (IFHRO), a core international curriculum has been developed for use in training coders. The curriculum provides a standard basis for education in all countries. A nine-module training course is recommended, as outlined below.

Module	Intent
1–Knowledge of basic medical science	To develop an understanding of the medical terminology that will be encountered in cause-of-death statements, of the structure and function of the human body, and of the nature of disease.
2–Legal and ethical issues relevant to the country in which coding is being conducted	To introduce the legal and ethical issues applicable to health information, its collection and release.
3–General use of underlying cause-of-death data	To explain the purpose for which underlying cause-of-death data are collected and how they are used.
4–Specific use of underlying-cause-of-death data	To introduce the specific use of coded mortality data.
5–Users of mortality data	To explain the different groups and stakeholders who are users of mortality data.
6–Sources of mortality data	To explain the roles of all the different people responsible for reporting data on the deceased, and the sources of that data.
7–The ICD	To develop an understanding of the ICD and to develop the knowledge and skills that are necessary to assign valid codes for cause of death.
8–How to code	To provide detailed instruction and practice on how to apply the coding rules and assign codes.
9–Quality assurance	To raise awareness of the various factors that influence the quality of coded data, and to describe techniques for ensuring the highest quality data possible.

Improving the quality and use of birth, death and cause-of-death information

The WHO assessment framework

Subcomponent D3: Quality of mortality coding

Having the right tools is vital for good coding. Coders should work from a copy of the three ICD volumes – *Tabular list*,[7] *Instruction manual* and *Alphabetical index* – to ensure proper code allocation. Many countries also use the ACME decision tables to help coders to select the correct underlying cause. Use of these tools also ensures that all coders consistently assign the same code to the terms used on the death certificates.

- **D3.1** Do all coders have a complete set of ICD volumes available to them when they code?
- **D3.2** Do all coders have a set of the ACME decisions tables?

Annual updates to the ICD codes and coding practices are determined by WHO-FIC and routinely posted on the WHO web site for the ICD. Keeping up-to-date with these revisions helps to ensure international comparability of the data.

- **D3.3** Do you regularly check:
  - the ICD web site[7] for updates to codes and coding practices?
  - the department of health's web site for updates on coding practices?

Poor coding practices detract from the utility of cause-of-death data and are a waste of resources. To ensure good quality coding, the work of coders should be systematically and periodically evaluated, to identify and correct any systematic errors or problems with coding practices.

- **D3.4** What processes are in place to assess the quality of cause of death coding, and how frequently is this assessed?
- **D3.5** Has the quality of mortality coding ever been evaluated?
- **D3.6** If so, was the level of accuracy deemed satisfactory? What systemic issues were identified?
- **D3.7** What mechanisms are in place to provide feedback to coders on the quality of coding, and to correct the problems and issues identified through evaluation and practice?

---

[7] http://www.who.int/classifications/icd/en/

3.7 Component E – Data access, use and quality checks

This section covers component E – *Data access, use and quality checks* – within which are the following subcomponents:

- E1 – Data quality and plausibility checks;
- E2 – Data tabulation;
- E3 – Data access and dissemination.

It is suggested that the subgroup that carries out the review of E1–E3 includes health analysts, demographers, statisticians and others involved with the analysis, compilation and dissemination of birth, death and cause-of-death data.

Data quality, access and use are critical components of any statistical system, but are often neglected. The result is that the information on births and deaths collected at great expense is not used as well as it could be, and those collecting the data are not fully rewarded for their efforts.

To be useful for public health and population-planning needs, data at the individual level need to be aggregated in a way that maximizes their public health relevance. There are international standards for the most useful ways of aggregating and tabulating data, and these standards can assist countries in the use of statistics for health and social policy and planning. For example, the UN provides a minimal list of recommended characteristics for tabulating birth and death statistics (*1*). The ICD proposes four different condensed cause-of-death tabulation lists, and also provides recommended age groups (*27*). More recently, WHO has provided advice to countries about how to compile leading cause of death lists (*33*).

In countries with compulsory and universal recording of vital events, the national vital statistics system should be able to provide annual data showing frequency distributions for births, deaths and cause of death; geographical differentials for the most important characteristics; and time series showing the major trends (at least over the past decade or two). However, the full utility of vital statistics will only become clear to government planners if the statistics are compiled and presented in ways that are understandable to non-statisticians. Policy-makers are constantly searching for evidence that can be incorporated into decision-making processes about population health priorities. The value of the data for most public health purposes will be much greater and more meaningful if tabulations of frequencies are converted into birth and death *rates*, and causes of death are compiled and ranked according to *leading causes* of deaths.

Death rates will be of much greater public health use if they are calculated separately for different age groups (usually 5-year age groups up to at least age 85 years and over, but preferably to age 100 years and over). There are strong epidemiological justifications for this. The causes of child deaths are very different to the causes of adult deaths. For instance, conditions common around the perinatal period (e.g. birth asphyxia and birth trauma) kill many infants but not adults, and pneumonia, diarrhoea and measles are more common causes of death in childhood than later in life. Conversely, adults are more likely than children to die from chronic diseases such as cancer or heart disease.

For some decision-makers and for some purposes, a single statistic that summarizes death rates over all ages, such as "life expectancy", may be preferable to their needs. Death rates are usually age standardized, to separate the impact of population age structure from true mortality impact. There are guidelines on how to choose a standard age structure to determine "age-standardized rates", as well as advice on how to calculate and interpret the results (*30*).

As with age, data and analyses of causes of death should always be presented separately for males and females, to maximize their public health value. Some causes of death (e.g. road traffic accidents) are more common among men than women. Conversely, only women can die from maternal causes, and some cancers (e.g.

The WHO assessment framework

cervical cancer in women and prostate cancer in men) are clearly sex-specific.

When reviewing the way that data are tabulated, it is important to ensure that transparent and well-documented procedures are used to calculate vital rates and other indicators, and that this information is included with the data. For example, when converting the death statistics into "mortality rates", care should be taken that general population data (denominators) accurately reflect the population from which the number of deaths (numerators) were recorded. One common error is to include deaths from non-residents in the numerator, but not in the resident population at risk of dying (denominator). Non-resident deaths would normally be excluded from the numerator, because the purpose of calculating such rates is to accurately reflect the risk of death in the resident population that is the focus of public policy responses. Conversely, in epidemiological surveillance systems, particularly for the control of disease outbreaks, all deaths should be included wherever they occur, and irrespective of resident status.

While civil registration is the most important source of data on fertility and mortality levels, it is not the only source. Typically, countries (usually the national statistics office) will have carried out a number of censuses and surveys. In many cases, these will have included questions about vital events occurring in the population, from which levels of fertility and mortality, by age and sex, can be estimated. Demographers have developed several methods to estimate mortality and fertility from censuses and surveys, and these estimates should be *routinely* compared with the levels of age-specific and sex-specific mortality and fertility calculated from vital registration. Typically, vital rates from censuses and surveys are higher than comparable rates from vital registration in countries where they are undertaken, suggesting an underreporting of deaths and births in the civil registration system (Box 3.8).

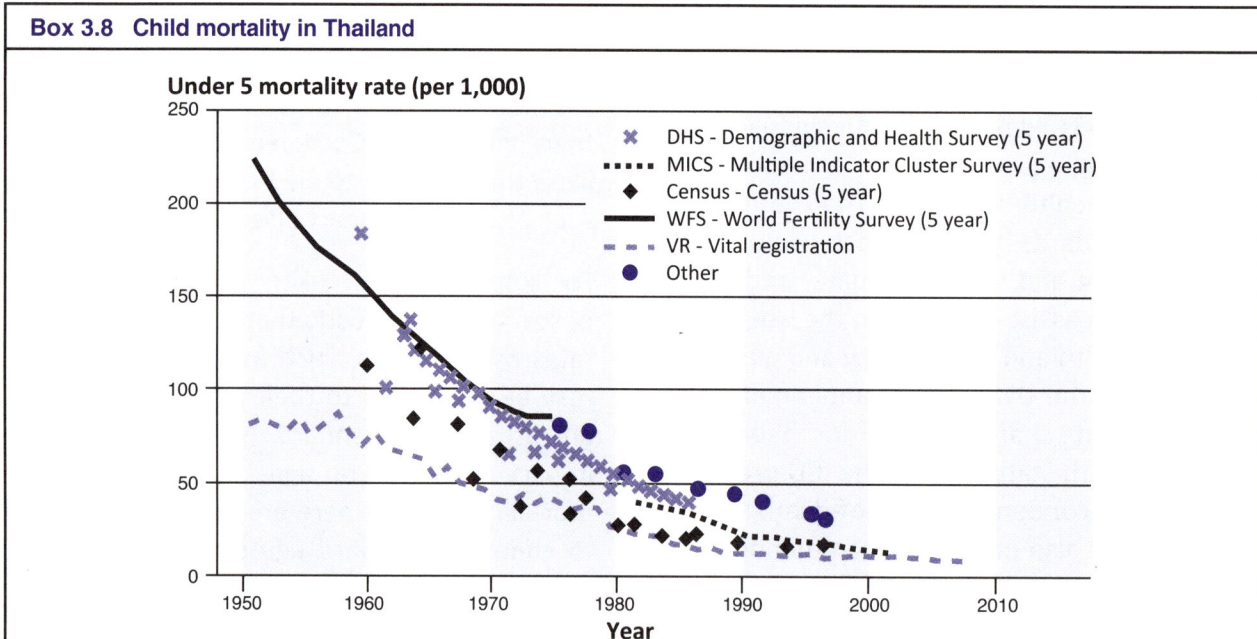

Box 3.8 Child mortality in Thailand

The graph shows how estimates of "child mortality" (i.e. death before age 5) in Thailand derived from censuses or surveys can be used to estimate the degree of underreporting of child deaths (completeness) in the vital registration system, and how this has changed over time. This is done by comparing the line of best "fit" for the observed child mortality rates derived from censuses and surveys in Thailand with the actual observed values calculated from vital registration data for the same year or years. From this analysis it can be concluded that child deaths were grossly underreported in the national vital registration system in the 1970s and 1980s. However, levels of reporting appear to have improved dramatically over the past decade.

Countries are strongly urged to prepare similar visual aids of the comparative levels of child mortality derived from difference sources as critical background information about the performance of their death registration system.

In the case of cause-of-death statistics, tabulating and checking the validity of data is more complex. Before data are released, a number of simple plausibility and consistency checks should always be performed to assess how robust and credible the data are, and for what purpose they can be used. For example, an important consideration in assessing the quality of cause-of-death statistics is the need to identify and analyse the proportion of deaths that have been assigned to ill-defined cause-of-death categories. This proportion should be carefully monitored over time, because any change in the proportion of deaths assigned to these categories will affect the interpretation of trends in specific causes. Deaths coded to these categories have no public health utility, and great efforts should be made to avoid this practice. In discussing this problem, those participating in the assessment should ask whether the lack of specificity for those deaths coded to ill-defined causes is due to poor coding practices, poor certification, or both. This is important since the remedies for each will be different.

It is also important to be aware that some major cause-of-death categories in the ICD contain several non-specific disease codes that tend to be overused in countries with poor certification and coding. These "convenience" codes are also of very limited value for public health purposes. For example, within the broad category of cancers (malignant neoplasms) there is an ICD-10 cause-of-death code – C80 – that can be used when the primary site is unknown. This code is intended to be used only in exceptional cases when a doctor does not know the medical history of a patient or has no way of inferring the primary site from the cancer type. In some countries, up to 50% of cancer deaths are coded to this non-specific category with no indication given of the primary site. Such data are of very limited value in guiding cancer prevention efforts, because cancer control programmes vary enormously, depending on the primary site involved.

The same is true for the injury category – Chapter XIX of the ICD – which contains several codes that can be used when it is not clear what the injury was (which body part) or what caused it, or even whether it was accidental or intentional (suicide or homicide). Once again, injury deaths coded to these categories are of little value in guiding prevention efforts since widely different prevention strategies would need to be implemented, depending on the cause of injury and the degree of intent.

Perhaps most importantly, great care should be exercised to ensure that cardiovascular deaths are coded to specific conditions (such as ischaemic heart disease) instead of using vague convenience codes such as "heart failure" (code I50) or "cardiac arrhythmias" (code I49). If these codes are overused, the importance of ischaemic heart disease (for which prevention and treatment programmes are available) will be severely underestimated. Avoiding these vague and ill-defined diagnoses wherever possible requires additional care and appreciation among certifying doctors of the true value of accurate cause-of-death statistics.

Even when a specific cause of death is assigned, there is a need to be critical and ask whether the high frequency of a given cause is real, or is being influenced by diagnostic fashions. In many countries, there appear to be one or two vague terms that are grossly overused by certifying doctors, which can result in serious misinterpretation of the actual importance of different diseases and injuries. For example, in the United Kingdom "bronco-pneumonia" is used in this way, while in Russia, "myocardial degeneration" is commonly used to describe what are likely to be true cases of ischaemic heart disease.

Plausibility checks should also be carried out for causes of death for which alternative sources of data (other than vital registration) are available. For example, police records will usually contain data on deaths from traffic accidents, suicides and homicides. Cancer registries, as well as recording the incident (new) cases (for which they are primarily designed), may also record deaths from cancer, which could be checked against the cancer deaths included in vital registration (although in general, cancer registries are not good sources of mortality data). Confidential enquiries or other studies may also have been carried out to estimate maternal mortality. Every effort should be made to identify these alternative registers and

The WHO assessment framework

sources, and to compare the death rates derived from them to those recorded in the vital registration system for each cause of interest.

To obtain an overview of mortality patterns in a population, many countries find it useful to rank causes of death in order of their frequency and public health importance. The advantage of using a ranking method for causes of death is that it is based solely on the numbers of deaths, and no population denominator is required. Leading cause-of-death rankings can be produced for the entire population but are more meaningful if calculated separately for males and females, and for children and adults (as described above). Comparing the leading causes of death over time can also be used to check for data consistency; major changes from year to year are unlikely and should be investigated. Countries can also compare their national pattern of leading causes of death with those estimated by the WHO (see Annex D) for broad categories of countries at similar or different levels of socioeconomic development. Annex D provides information on distribution of leading causes of death by age and income groups. While these standard patterns will rarely apply exactly in any one country, they are nonetheless indicative of how causes of death change in importance with economic development and by age groups.

When comparing leading-cause distributions, it is vital to bear in mind that the way causes are grouped or split into subgroups will directly influence the rankings. Thus, before any conclusions are drawn, it is important to verify that the rankings that are being compared were obtained using the same condensed list of causes of death. If not, the ordering of leading causes will not be comparable. To help ensure comparability when ranking causes of death, WHO has proposed a standard list for use in deriving leading causes of death (*33*). The proposed list consists of 65 categories of disease and injury from which the 10 (or other selected number of) leading causes can be derived. The disease groupings have an epidemiological basis associated with control measures and have been tested for applicability in a broad range of countries. The list contains only one residual category ("all remaining causes") which, as with the ill-defined categories described above, should be excluded from the ranking. Other rankings of leading causes of death have also been proposed, such as that used in the Global Burden of Disease Study (*30*).

Another simple check on the epidemiological profile of a particular country is to verify that the first five leading causes of death account for 40–50% of deaths, while the first 10 leading causes should typically account for 55–65% of all *specified* deaths (i.e. deaths other than those coded to the residual and ill-defined categories mentioned above). An analysis of the leading causes of death is, however, only the starting point in the overall analysis of a national mortality profile. Supplementary analyses of the leading causes need to be undertaken, such as detailed cause-specific analysis. In particular, countries should calculate the age distribution of deaths from the 10 leading causes of death, and compare this to the distribution observed in a country or countries with good quality cause-of-death data. This will serve to verify that ages at death for leading causes are being correctly assigned and that improbable cause-of-death diagnoses at different ages are not common. If groupings of external causes appear among the leading causes it is particularly important that these are analysed in detail, for instance by using the injury matrix developed by the International Collaborative Effort on Injury Statistics (*34*). The ICD-10 injury mortality matrix organizes injury diagnoses for each type of external cause of death into meaningful groupings by body region and by nature of injury.

In conclusion, data evaluation and critical assessment should be an integral part of all vital statistics systems. A cost-effective way to do this is to use simple consistency and plausibility checks such as those proposed in subcomponent E1, and to regularly compare the data produced by the vital statistics system to information from other sources. Hence, it is essential for countries to know what other sources of information on fertility or mortality levels are available. Indeed, all existing sources, whether continuous or not, should be used to help evaluate the quality of the data produced by the vital registration system.

The WHO assessment framework

Subcomponent E1: Data quality and plausibility checks

Supporting material to be prepared in advance:

- Tabulations of relevant vital event data from other sources (e.g. censuses with birth and death questions, demographic and health surveys (DHS) and other national surveys). Calculations of birth and death rates from these sources compared with birth and death rates derived from civil registration (see Box 3.8).
- Calculations of the percentage distribution of deaths for the latest available year according to three broad cause-of-death groups I, II and III, as shown in Box 3.10.
- Calculations of the percentage distribution of deaths for the latest available year according to cause-of-death groups I, II and III within 5-year or 10-year age intervals (see Box 3.11).
- Calculation of the percentage of deaths by age and sex being assigned to ill-defined cause-of-death categories.

Subcomponent E1 (A): Levels of fertility and mortality

The best way to check the plausibility of vital statistics is to convert them into birth and death rates or ratios. Consistency checks should always be carried out both on the raw data and on key indicators (e.g. birth and death rates) before they are used or made more widely available. This can be done simply by comparing the raw data, and the rates derived from them, to corresponding figures from previous years. Major changes in numbers or rates are unlikely from year to year and should be investigated.

E1.1 Are fertility indicators (e.g. crude birth or fertility rate, age-specific fertility rate and total fertility rate) routinely calculated from the civil registration and vital statistics data?

E1.2 If so, which indicators are calculated?

E1.3 Are mortality indicators (e.g. crude death or mortality rate, age-specific mortality rate, infant mortality rate, neonatal mortality rate and maternal mortality rate) routinely calculated from the civil registration and vital statistics data?

E1.4 If so, which indicators are calculated?

E1.5 What data sources are used as the denominators to calculate these rates?

E1.6 Describe the plausibility and consistency checks that are carried out on the data and indicators before they are released for use (see Box 3.9).

It should not be assumed that, just because a country has a vital statistics system, the data the country produces are accurate. There are many potential sources of error in the vital statistics, including underregistration, age misreporting of deaths, and incorrect certification and coding of the underlying cause of death. Therefore, countries should carry out a range of consistency checks to identify possible sources of error in the data. This knowledge (e.g. about underregistration of deaths) will guide efforts to redress the problems.

E1.7 Are the civil registration and vital statistics data used to investigate variations in fertility and mortality within the country? If so, describe how this is being done.

E1.8 Are fertility rates derived from civil registration and vital statistics compared with rates derived from other sources?

E1.9 Are mortality rates derived from civil registration and vital statistics compared with rates derived from other sources?

Improving the quality and use of birth, death and cause-of-death information

The WHO assessment framework

> **Subcomponent E1 (A): Levels of fertility and mortality (cont.)**
>
> In countries lacking reliable vital statistics systems the investigation of fertility and mortality is particularly important. If the completeness of vital registration data is less than about 90%, the UN advises countries to include both fertility and mortality questions in the census. Estimates of fertility and mortality derived from census data, however, are approximate and subject to various errors, and should be adjusted using standard demographic techniques (*19*). Nonetheless, these data can be useful for estimating the completeness and overall performance of vital registration.
>
> E1.10 Did the last census include a question on births or deaths; for example:
> - Number of children ever born alive and still alive?
> - Date of birth of last child born alive?
> - Whether the last birth was registered?
> - Whether the last death was registered?
> - Deaths in the household in the past 12–24 months?
>
> E1.11 If so, have the data been analysed and compared with the vital statistics data?
>
> Other sources (e.g. church, cemetery, police, village records and different administrative databases) can be used to complete and verify vital registration data, through matching of births and deaths.
>
> E1.12 Are other sources used to complete and verify birth and death data?
>
> E1.13 If so, describe these.

Box 3.9 Standard plausibility and consistency checks

It is useful to carry out standard plausibility or consistency checks on the vital statistics by combining or aggregating the data into standard 5-year age groups. For fertility, births should be grouped according to age of mother, namely <15 years, 15–19 years, 20–24 years, ... , 45–49 years and 50+ years.

For mortality, deaths should be aggregated into the following age groups: <1 year (i.e. died before reaching the first birthday), 1–4 years, 5–9 years, 10–14 years, ... , 80–84 years and 85+ years. Wherever possible, deaths should be tabulated up to age 100 in 5-year age groups.

Age-specific fertility rates (for ages of the mother shown above) and age-specific mortality rates (for the ages at death shown above) should be calculated separately for males and females. An estimate of the mid-year population by age and sex is required to calculate the rates.

Based on these aggregate numbers of deaths (and births) by age, and on the age-specific birth and death rates, countries should calculate the metrics listed below from their vital statistics data, and should carefully review their findings to make a preliminary assessment of the quality of their vital statistics data.

Calculate the ratio of male births ($B(m)$) to female births ($B(f)$). This ratio should be about 1.05. Significant departures indicate underreporting of births for either males or females, with the latter being the more likely. The pattern of age-specific fertility rates should show a peak level for women aged 25–29 or 30–34 years, and decline thereafter.

Calculate the crude death rate (reported deaths × 1000/total population size). The rate should be about 5–10 per 1000. Crude death rates below 5 per 1000 should be viewed with suspicion. (Note: the crude death rate should not vary by more than about 3–5% each year. Annual variations greater than this amount should be investigated.)

Plot the log of the age-specific death rate at each age. The graph should show a high rate at ages 1 year and 1–4 years, a trough at ages 5–14 years, a small bump at ages 15–34 years (due to accidents in males, and to maternal mortality and accidents in females), and a consistent increase (seen as a straight line) from about the age of 35 years onwards. Departures from this linear trend with age suggest underreporting or misreporting of age at death.

For comparisons of fertility and mortality rates within and between countries, it is important to standardize for differences in age distributions (*24*).[8]

All opportunities should be used to further check the plausibility of the vital statistics data, by comparing the fertility and mortality rates from civil registration data with those derived from other sources. Major differences in rates or ratios should be investigated. Rates derived from other sources (such as DHS or UNICEF's multiple indicator cluster surveys (MICS) or some other health or demographic survey) should be used as comparators (see Box 3.8).

---

[8] See www.who.int/healthinfo/paper31.pdf

The WHO assessment framework

Subcomponent E1 (B): Cause of death

A frequently used indicator of the quality of cause-of-death data is the percentage of all deaths for which the cause is classified as ill-defined (Chapter XVIII of the ICD-10). Ill-defined causes are of no public health value. Also, where they are common, they will make the cause-of-death distribution unreliable, because true causes of death are hidden and hence underestimated. Generally, the percentage of deaths for which the cause is ill-defined should be less than 10% at ages 65 years and over, and less than 5% at ages below 65 years.

If the percentage of ill-defined causes has declined significantly, caution must be exercised when interpreting trends in specific causes (such as cancers or heart disease), because changes in death rates from these causes may be largely or entirely due to a redistribution effect from ill-defined to more-specific causes.

The need to reduce ill-defined causes of death should not force the certifying doctor to give a defined cause in all instances: there will inevitably be occasions when a cause of death cannot be indicated with precision. Such, "unknown" causes (code R99) should be measured and tabulated separately, and should not constitute more than about 2–3% of all deaths.

- **E1.14** What is the proportion of all deaths allocated to ill-defined categories? (See Annex 1 of Volume 2 of ICD-10 and Section 4.1.10 of ICD-10, Rule A on *Senility and other ill-defined conditions*.)
- **E1.15** Has the proportion of deaths allocated to the ill-defined categories changed over time?
- **E1.16** What is the proportion of unknown causes of death among all deaths?

Apart from exceptional cases (e.g. HIV/AIDS or other high-mortality epidemics), national cause-of-death patterns do not change significantly in the short term. Simple percentage distributions of deaths by cause will reveal unexpected deviations in patterns of causes of death that should be further investigated. Breaks in series due to ICD version changes may also cause variations, and need to be noted. There is little that can be done to correct for discontinuities caused by changes to the ICD other than conducting in-depth comparability studies, but care should be exercised when interpreting such changes because they are unlikely to be due to real increases (or decreases) in disease rates.

Checking the annual numbers of deaths assigned to specific causes can be sufficient to identify major changes in the use of cause-of-death categories from one year to another. Such changes should not occur without a good reason (e.g. a natural disaster) and should be investigated.

It is also important to carry out this consistency check at different levels of data aggregation, particularly for major administrative groups of the country. This will enable users to detect whether the quality of reporting at a local level has changed from one year to another. If so, this should be investigated.

- **E1.17** Is the consistency of the national cause-of-death pattern checked over time, including disaggregation comparisons?

There is a close and predictable relationship between causes of death and life expectancy, which has been validated by long time-series from many different settings. As life expectancy increases, the proportion of communicable, maternal and perinatal causes decreases, while the proportion of noncommunicable diseases (such as heart disease and cancer) increases. These relationships should be used to check the plausibility of the cause-of-death pattern provided by the vital statistics system.

- **E1.18** Does the overall cause-of-death distribution seems plausible, e.g. does it fit the expected disease and injury patterns given current national levels of life expectancy (see Box 3.10)?

Broad causes of death, such as communicable or noncommunicable diseases and injuries, show a predictable pattern at different ages. Significant departures from this pattern suggest problems with the quality of vital statistics and can be used to check for plausibility.

- **E1.19** Is the age pattern of causes of death obtained from civil registration for major disease groups and injuries consistent with expected patterns? (see Box 3.11)

Improving the quality and use of birth, death and cause-of-death information

The WHO assessment framework

> **Subcomponent E1 (B): Cause of death (cont.)**
>
> It is common for deaths to be certified to vague causes within broad-cause categories. For example, a death may be certified as due to heart failure, arteriosclerosis or some other vague diagnosis. Cancer deaths may be certified to an ill-defined primary site of cancer or to no specified primary site. Understanding the dimensions of such certification practices is important. Both certifying doctors and coders frequently use the three categories referred to below in E.1.20, but they are of limited public health value. In such circumstances, it is important to consult the patient records or to check with the treating physician, to obtain additional information that can be used to correctly certify and code the death.
>
> **E1.20 Further checks on the quality of cause-of-death data can be made using the three measures below. In properly functioning systems with good death certification, the percentage of all cardiovascular, cancer or injury deaths assigned to these codes should not exceed about 10–15%.**
>
> - **What is the proportion of cardiovascular disease deaths assigned to heart failure and other ill-defined heart-disease categories (ICD-10 codes I472, I490, I46, I50, I514, I515, I516, I519, I709)?**
> - **What is the proportion of cancers with an ill-defined primary site (ICD-10 codes C76, C80, C97)?**
> - **What is the proportion of injury deaths that are of undetermined intent (ICD-10 codes Y10-Y34, Y872)?**

Box 3.10   Percent of deaths expected from three broad cause-of-death groups (I–III) as a function of increases in life expectancy

Life Expectancy (years)	Broad cause-of-death groups			
	Group I (%)	Group II (%)	Group III (%)	Total (%)
55	22	65	13	100
60	16	70	14	100
65	13	74	13	100
70	11	78	11	100

Group I: Communicable diseases, maternal, perinatal and nutritional conditions (ICD-10 codes A00–B99, G00–G04, N70–N73, J00–J06, J10–J18, J20–J22, H65–H66, O00–O99, P00–P96, E00–E02, E40–E46, E50, D50–D53, D64.9, E51–64)

Group II: Noncommunicable diseases (ICD-10 codes C00–C97, D00–D48, D55–D64 (minus D 64.9) D65–D89, E03–E07, E10–E16, E20–E34, E65–E88, F01–F99, G06–G98, H00–H61, H68–H93, I00–I99, J3–J98, K00–K92, N00–N64, N75–N98, L00–L98, M00–M99, Q00–Q99)

Group III: Intentional and non-intentional injuries (including homicide and suicide)(ICD-10 codes V01–Y89)

The table above shows how the relative importance of different broad causes of death changes as the average life expectancy of a population increases. Three broad cause groups are shown:

- Group I – Infectious and parasitic diseases, maternal and perinatal and nutritional causes.
- Group II – Cancers, heart disease, stroke, chronic lung, liver and other noncommunicable diseases, and mental health conditions such as schizophrenia.
- Group III – Injuries, such as accidents, homicides and suicides.

At each level of life expectancy, the typical distribution (as a percentage) of deaths that one might expect to find is shown in the table above. For example, a country with an average life expectancy of 55 years would typically have about 22% of deaths due to group I diseases, and about 65% due to group 2 (i.e. noncommunicable diseases such as cancer, heart disease and stroke). A country with lower mortality and higher life expectancy (e.g. 65 years) would expect a smaller percentage of deaths from group I causes (13%) and a higher percentage from group II causes (74%). In other words, as the life expectancy in a country improves, the relative importance (percentage of deaths) of group I diseases declines, due to better infectious diseases control; hence, more people can be expected to die from noncommunicable diseases or even injuries.

In using this table, first situate the country according to the most recent life expectancy estimates, then interpolate between the percentage distributions in the table to estimate the expected percentage of deaths from groups I, II and III. The expected distribution should be compared to the observed distribution of deaths as calculated from the vital statistics to determine the plausibility of the observed cause-of-death pattern across the three groups. All ill-defined causes should be ignored when making comparisons.

The WHO assessment framework

Box 3.11 Typical age pattern of board cause-of-death groups (I–III)

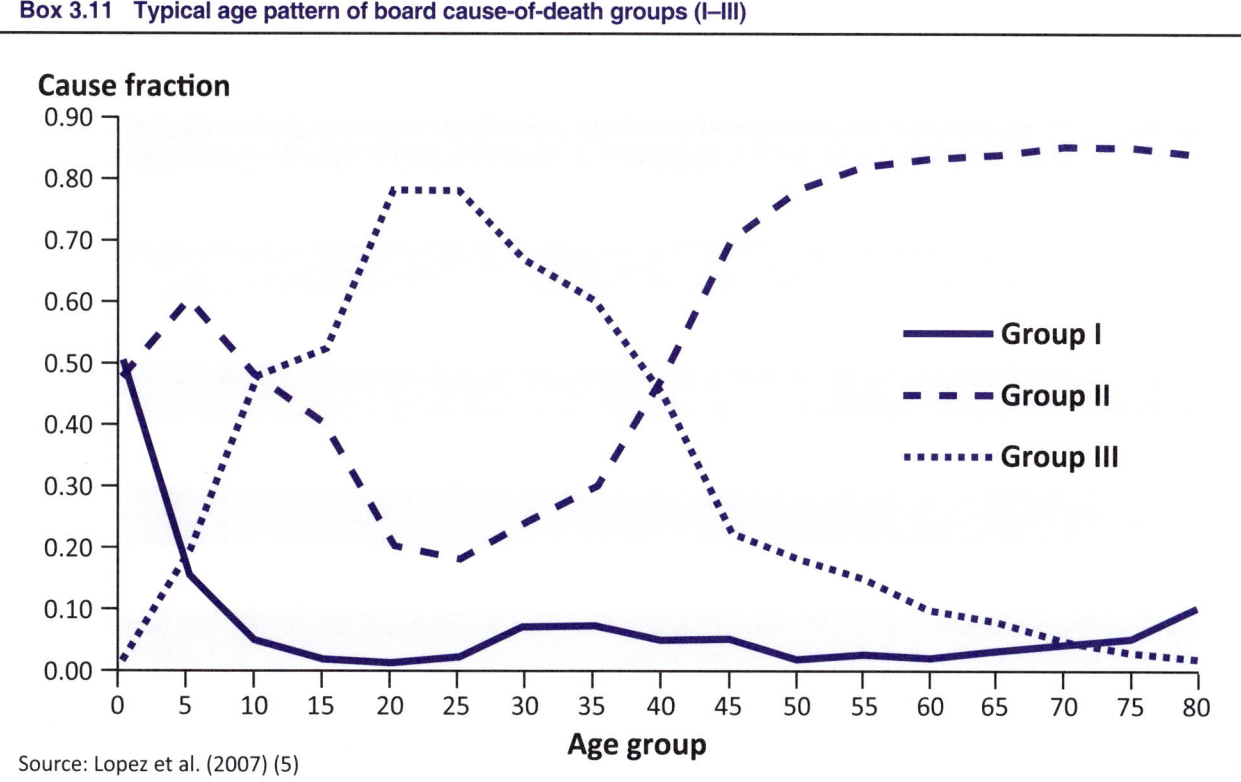

Source: Lopez et al. (2007) (5)

The chart shows the typical age distribution of deaths for the three broad groups of causes described in Box 3.10:

- Group I – Communicable diseases, maternal, perinatal and nutritional conditions.
- Group II – Noncommunicable diseases.
- Group III – Intentional and non-intentional injuries, including homicide and suicide.

The chart shows a hypothetical example of a country with a life expectancy of 65 years. The typical percentage distribution of causes at each age would be similar at other levels of life expectancy between about 55 and 75 years. Comparing this typical pattern with the age and cause distribution generated from the vital statistics system permits a plausibility check of the age pattern of causes of death.

In conducting plausibility checks of the age pattern of causes of death, the first step is to compute the distribution of deaths across the three broad cause groups for deaths within each age group: <1 year, 1–4 years, 5–9 years, 10–14 years, … , 80–84 years, 85+ years. The next step is to plot the cause fractions (i.e. percentage deaths from each broad cause group) for each age group, to produce a chart similar to the example shown above.

Separate charts should be computed for male deaths and female deaths, although in the absence of high maternal mortality rates, the cause fractions by age for the sexes should be similar. Typically, about half to two thirds of all deaths at ages <5 years are due to group I causes, particularly infectious diseases and pneumonia, and other communicable diseases such as malaria. Perinatal conditions such as birth trauma and birth asphyxia are also common causes at these ages, whereas injuries (particularly accidents) are not. Injuries become progressively more important a cause of death in older children and young adults, so that by about age 20–24 years, typically 70–80% of all deaths are due to accidents, homicide or suicide. The cause-specific fractions from injuries for females at these ages are typically slightly lower than for males. Beyond age 40 years, the percentage of deaths due to group II (noncommunicable) diseases rises sharply, so that by about age 60 years, they typically account for about 80% of deaths. There may be a slight decline in the cause fraction of group II diseases at ages above 80 years due to the importance of pneumonia (a group I disease) as a cause of death in the elderly.

The chart shows a hypothetical example of a typical cause-of-death pattern at different ages. The precise distribution of causes will, of course, vary from country to country. However, significant departures from this age pattern should be closely investigated because they would be suggestive of problems with either the certification and coding of causes of death, or age-misreporting of deaths, or both.

While country age patterns of causes of death should be broadly similar to the hypothetical example shown in the chart, important exceptions may occur. For example, pandemic influenza deaths, generalized HIV epidemics, wars or natural disasters such as earthquakes or tsunamis may result in legitimate and understandable departures from these typical age patterns for one or more years. What is important is an understanding of the reasons for any deviations from this typical age pattern of cause-of-death distribution.

Note that the figures do not include deaths due to ill-defined causes.

Improving the quality and use of birth, death and cause-of-death information

The WHO assessment framework

Subcomponent E2: Data tabulation

The UN recommends that vital statistics be compiled according to date of occurrence. However, in many countries, birth and death statistics are compiled according to date of registration because this is simpler than re-allocating events to the year of occurrence. Vital statistics tabulated by date of registration can be misleading, particularly if a large number of delayed births and deaths are registered as a result of periodic registration campaigns.

E2.1 Are births and deaths compiled according to date of occurrence or to date of registration?

Place of occurrence is usually the geographical location (locality/town) where the birth or death took place. For policy and services planning, it is also important to know the place of usual residence of the parents, or of the deceased in case of death registration.

E2.2 Are births and deaths compiled according to place of occurrence as well as place of usual residence?

All mortality data should be tabulated separately by age, sex and underlying cause of death. The probability of dying varies substantially at different ages for men and women but can also vary substantially within a country between different regions. Each country should decide what geographic disaggregation of birth and death statistics is appropriate for its policy and planning needs.

E2.3 At what level of disaggregation are the birth data tabulated? Report separately for:
- sex;
- sex, and age of mother;
- sex, age of mother and subregion.

E2.4 At what level of disaggregation are the deaths and cause-of-death data tabulated? Report separately for deaths and cause of death for:
- sex;
- sex and age;
- sex and subregion;
- sex, age and subregion.

The risk of death varies significantly by age, and death statistics should always be complied according to the age at which death occurred. Countries should use the WHO standard age groupings to do this.

E2.5 Are standard WHO age groups used to tabulate mortality and cause-of-death data?

Subnational tabulations are important for revealing geographical inequalities in heath status with implications for health-services planning.

E2.6 What is the smallest subnational level used for tabulating vital statistics? Is this appropriate given the potential uses for disaggregated data?

Standard tabulation lists are useful for comparing trends in diseases and health status across different populations and time periods.[9] WHO requests countries to report data according to the four-character ICD level.

E2.7 Are any of the four standard mortality tabulation lists suggested by the ICD used for data presentation purposes?

E2.8 If not, which condensed list is used? How was this list derived?

---

[9] See ICD-10: http://www.who.int/classifications/icd/ICD-10_2nd_ed_volume2.pdf

The WHO assessment framework

Subcomponent E2: Data tabulation (cont.)

Public health authorities usually want information on the diseases that cause the most premature deaths. Statistics on leading causes of death should always be shown separately for men and women.

The level of disaggregation used for the cause-of-death database will influence the ranking of selected diseases and injuries. Comparisons between countries should only be made using comparable ranking lists.

Ill-defined causes should not be included when ranking causes of death but shown separately and not included with the residual or other causes category.

Some countries include deaths of nationals currently residing outside the country who die overseas in tabulations. If this is the current practice, these deaths and all nationals should be included in the national population estimates when calculating rates.

- **E2.9** Are data compiled into 10 leading causes (separately for men and women and children)?
- **E2.10** From which list are the 10 leading causes selected?
- **E2.11** Are ill-defined causes included in the ranking as a category?
- **E2.12** What proportion of deaths is accounted for by the 10 leading causes of death?

Subcomponent E3: Data access and dissemination

Supplementary material to be prepared in advance:

- Compile a list of publications and information products available that use the vital statistics.

The main data users should be involved in determining the most appropriate cross tabulations and regional breakdowns of the vital statistics data that are relevant to their needs. It is important to solicit feedback from users about the relevance, utility and quality of vital statistics. There is little point in producing data that are not used, or are regarded as unnecessary.

- **E3.1** Who are the main users of the vital statistics:
  - within government?
  - outside the government?
- **E3.2** Is there an engagement strategy to regularly discuss data needs with the main data users? If so, describe this.
- **E3.3** Is it possible to provide an example of how vital statistics have been used to guide policy and practice?

Timeliness of data is one of the quality criteria that users rate most highly. This is particularly important for local-level and small-area data. Data-release dates are important both for producers and users. Keeping to release dates allows users to plan their work around availability of vital statistics.

Understanding of vital statistics can be facilitated by issuing brief analytical reports based on the data. For example, reports that give a brief account of significant changes in mortality levels, or differences by sex, or trends in leading causes of death are extremely useful. The principal purpose of such reports is to summarize the key messages from the vital statistics for policy use.

- **E3.4** What is the time from the end of the reporting period (e.g. end of calendar year in which births and deaths occurred) to the dissemination of:
  - birth and death statistics?
  - cause-of-death statistics?
- **E3.5** Are analytical reports about birth, deaths and causes of deaths derived from vital registration produced? If so, include examples.
- **E3.6** Is there a data-release schedule?

Improving the quality and use of birth, death and cause-of-death information

The WHO assessment framework

Subcomponent E3: Data access and dissemination (cont.)

To be useful, data have to be accessible to as many legitimate users as possible, preferably in both print and electronic form. Every effort should also be made to ensure that data are available to users at minimal cost. The more the data are used, the more feedback will be received about their quality.

- E3.7 Are vital statistics made available to users as:
  - print?
  - electronic files?
  - web sites?
  - pdfs?
  - interactive tables?
- E3.8 Are the vital statistics available free of charge or at a cost? Please explain.

Official vital statistics should be published annually by a trustworthy government source. The correct use and understanding of the data depends on supplying information about the data ("metadata") along with the data themselves. These metadata ensure that the data are interpreted appropriately by the end users.

- E3.9 What agency publishes the official vital statistics?
- E3.10 How regularly are the data published or released?
- E3.11 Are all definitions and concepts used in vital statistics publications clearly explained?

It is important for producers of the data to also be users of the data. As well as building essential analytical capacity (and providing quality checks), producers who are also users will help to build the case for improving the quality of vital statistics as their potential value will be better appreciated by those who collect them.

- E3.12 What analyses are being routinely carried out on the data (e.g. fertility patterns, mortality differentials, disease mapping, etc.)?
- E3.13 Along with the statistical tables, are analyses of the data published regularly?
- E3.14 How are these data being used at various levels?
- E3.15 Is there any attempt to build analytical capacity among staff who collect and compile vital statistics to perform basic analyses of the data to help them better understand the value and purpose of the data which they collect? If not, how could this be achieved?

Annex A Strategic planning for strengthening the vital statistics system

The steps required for preparing a strategic plan for strengthening the civil registration and vital statistics systems are described in Figure A1. It is important to ensure that the strategic plan is:

- part of the overall efforts that countries are undertaking to improve their health information system;
- aligned with and building on current efforts to strengthen the national statistical information system.

Figure A1 outlines the process and the main elements of the roadmap for carrying out the review of a country's civil registration and vital statistics systems, and divides it into the three standard phases commonly used for planning. These are further described in Chapter 2.

Figure A1 Process for preparing a plan to strengthen the vital statistics system

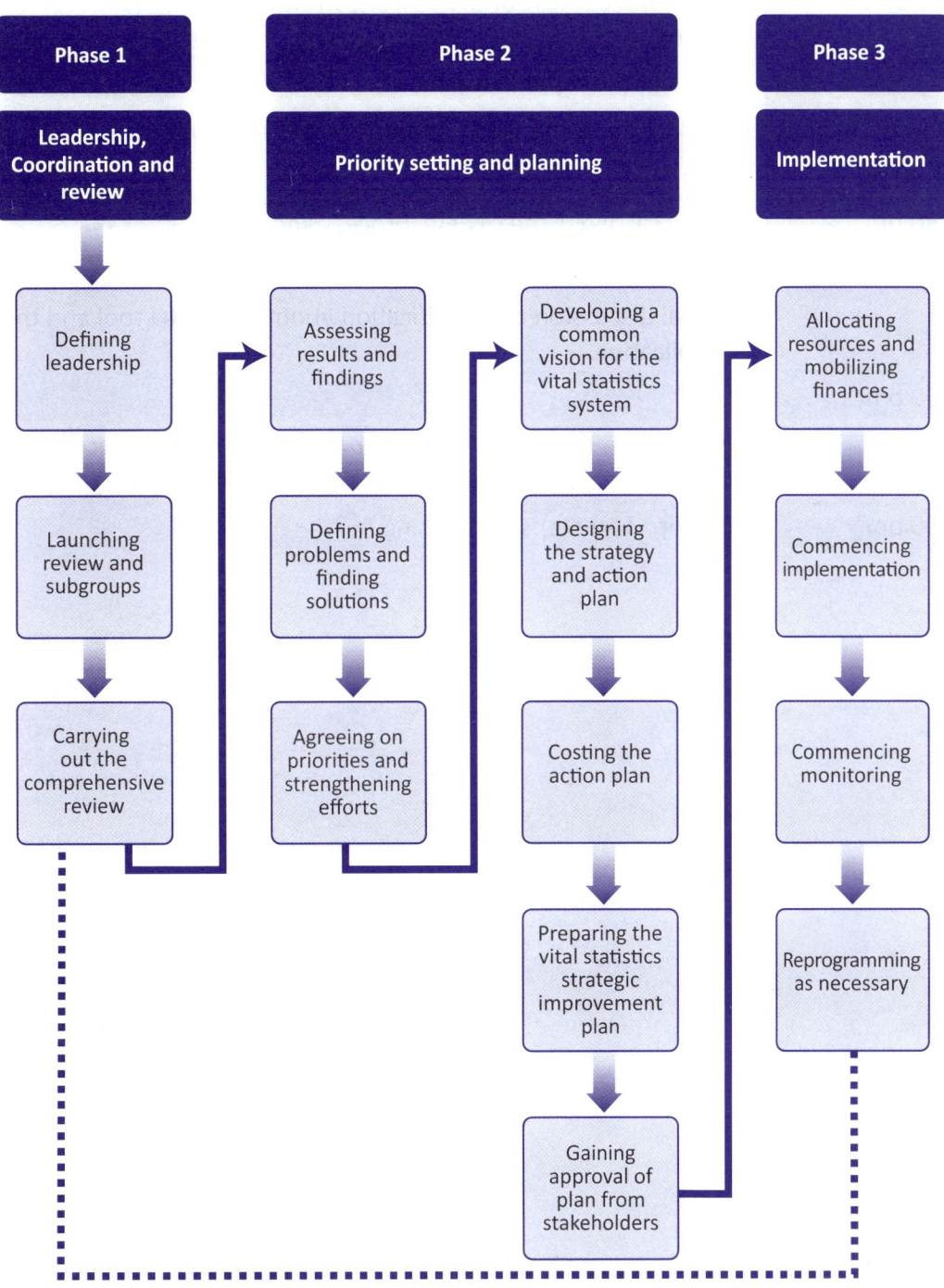

Improving the quality and use of birth, death and cause-of-death information 65

Annex B Template for launch meeting agenda

The template is an example of an agenda that was used for the first stakeholder meeting that launched the review of the civil registration and vital statistics systems.

Time	Agenda
8:30 – 9:00 am	Registration
9:00 – 9:30 am	Welcome/Opening remarks Plan for the day and agenda
9:30 – 10:00 am	Keynote address: Benefits of good vital statistics for local and national government authorities
10:00 – 10:30 am	Break
10:30 – 11:30 am	History and context of the civil registration and vital statistics in the country Results of the rapid assessment
11:30 am – 12:30 pm	Introduction to the WHO framework and review tool
12:30 – 1:30 pm	Lunch
1:30 – 2:30 pm	How to carry out the review: process and output
2:30 – 3:30 pm	Formation of subgroups General discussion and clarification about the WHO tool and the process of application
3:30 – 4:00 pm	Break
4:00 – 4:45 pm	Discussion in subgroups to further clarify the review process and subject matter(facilitated by members of the review committee)
4:45 – 5:00 pm	Wrap up, next steps and closing

Annex C Suggested indicators for monitoring progress in national civil registration and vital statistics systems

Any improvement process or implementation plan needs to be monitored to ensure that goals will be reached; it is therefore important to define a short list of indicators for monitoring progress (see Chapter 2 and Annex A). Some potential indicators are listed below, but each country will have to identify the core indicators that are most likely to reflect progress in their specific areas of concern. The selection of indicators should be based on explicit criteria such as relevance, measurability, understandability, responsiveness to change and data availability.

A database of core indicators – including baseline measures and related metadata – should be established and made publicly available, and progress should be reported at regular intervals. Monitoring reports should include the quantitative values for the indicators, as well as some analysis of the qualitative information. Documentation of progress will help to generate continuing support for the improvement plan, and additional funding from national or external sources.

Monitoring need not be onerous if it is planned for from the beginning; only a subset of the suggested indicators in table C1 needs to be selected. Some of the indicators may already exist and may already be in use for the annual reviews of the health sector.

Table C1 Suggested indicators

Aspect	Areas covered
Inputs	■ Budgets of the civil registration and vital statistics systems ■ Human resource component of these budgets ■ Number of staff doing registration duties
Processes	■ Access to civil registration (see Box 3.3 in main text) ■ Availability of civil registration (number of registration points) ■ Number and percentage of hospitals with registrars in situ ■ Completeness of birth registration, nationally and by region ■ Completeness of death registration, nationally and by region ■ Medically certified deaths as a percentage of total deaths annually ■ Number and percentage of civil registration points that report late (i.e. after scheduled date) ■ Percentage of all registration offices linked by computers to central level
Outputs	■ Time lag between data collection and publications (years) ■ Number of tables provided to the UN Demographic Yearbook (the UN asks countries to provide 30 tables on fertility and mortality for this publication) ■ Ill-defined causes of death as a percentage of all deaths annually ■ Cancer deaths assigned to ill-defined site as a percentage of all cancer deaths annually ■ Cardiovascular deaths assigned to ill-defined causes as a percentage of all cardiovascular deaths annually ■ Injury deaths assigned to undetermined causes as a percentage of all injury deaths ■ Infections and parasitic disease deaths assigned to septicaemia as a percentage of all infectious and parasitic deaths

Annex D Leading cause of deaths by age group and income group for both sexes

The four tables that show the 10 leading causes for some major age groups, and for high, middle and low-income countries, have been generated by WHO from their cause-specific mortality database. It is suggested that countries compare their own distribution of leading causes for all ages to the table for the income standard that most closely resembles their own. Major differences should be investigated further by comparing the leading causes for the four age groups – 0–9 years, 10–19 years, 20–59 years, and 60 years and over – to the provided standards.

Table D1 All ages

World

Rank	Cause	Deaths (000s)	%
1	Ischaemic heart disease	7195	12.2
2	Cerebrovascular disease	5710	9.7
3	Lower respiratory infections	4175	7.1
4	Chronic obstructive pulmonary disease	3024	5.1
5	Diarrhoeal diseases	2162	3.7
6	HIV	2038	3.5
7	Tuberculosis	1463	2.5
8	Trachea, bronchus and lung cancers	1323	2.3
9	Road traffic accidents	1274	2.2
10	Prematurity and low birth weight	1179	2.0

Low Income

Rank	Cause	Deaths (000s)	%
1	Lower respiratory infections	2906	11.2
2	Ischaemic heart disease	2432	9.4
3	Diarrhoeal diseases	1782	6.9
4	Cerebrovascular disease	1457	5.6
5	HIV/AIDS	1445	5.6
6	Chronic obstructive pulmonary disease	932	3.6
7	Tuberculosis	900	3.5
8	Neonatal infections[a]	889	3.4
9	Prematurity and low birth weight	836	3.2
10	Malaria	829	3.2

Middle Income

Rank	Cause	Deaths (000s)	%
1	Cerebrovascular disease	3474	14.1
2	Ischaemic heart disease	3397	13.8
3	Chronic obstructive pulmonary disease	1803	7.3
4	Lower respiratory infections	958	3.9
5	Trachea, bronchus and lung cancers	690	2.8
6	Road traffic accidents	679	2.8
7	Hypertensive disease	618	2.5
8	HIV/AIDS lung cancers	571	2.3
9	Tuberculosis	548	2.2
10	Stomach cancer	1179	2.2

High Income

Rank	Cause	Deaths (000s)	%
1	Ischaemic heart disease	1366	16.5
2	Cerebrovascular disease	778	9.4
3	Trachea, bronchus and lung cancers	484	5.8
4	Lower respiratory infections	310	3.7
5	Chronic obstructive pulmonary disease	289	3.5
6	Alzheimer and other dementias	278	3.4
7	Colon and rectum cancers	271	3.3
8	Diabetes mellitus	228	2.8
9	Breast cancer	164	2.0
10	Hypertensive disease	147	1.8

AIDS, acquired immunodeficiency syndrome; HIV, human immunodeficiency virus
[a] Includes severe neonatal infections and other non-infectious causes arising in the perinatal period.
Source: WHO (2004) (27)

Table D2 Ages 0–9 years

World

Rank	Cause	Deaths (000s)	%
1	Lower respiratory infections	1958	17.3
2	Diarrhoeal diseases	1789	15.8
3	Prematurity and low birth weight	1179	10.4
4	Neonatal infections[a]	1144	10.1
5	Birth asphyxia and birth trauma	856	7.6
6	Malaria	817	7.2
7	Measles	418	3.7
8	Congenital anomalies	382	3.4
9	HIV/AIDS	279	2.5
10	Pertussis	254	2.2

Low Income

Rank	Cause	Deaths (000s)	%
1	Lower respiratory infections	1666	18.7
2	Diarrhoeal diseases	1501	16.9
3	Neonatal infections[a]	889	10.0
4	Prematurity and low birth weight	836	9.4
5	Malaria	766	8.6
6	Birth asphyxia and birth trauma	648	7.3
7	Measles	388	4.4
8	Pertussis	240	2.7
9	Congenital anomalies	230	2.6
10	HIV/AIDS	218	2.4

Middle Income

Rank	Cause	Deaths (000s)	%
1	Prematurity and low birth weight	326	14.2
2	Lower respiratory infections	288	12.5
3	Diarrhoeal diseases	285	12.4
4	Neonatal infections[a]	241	10.5
5	Birth asphyxia and birth trauma	201	8.7
6	Congenital anomalies	132	5.7
7	HIV/AIDS	61	2.7
8	Malaria	52	2.2
9	Drownings	49	2.1
10	Meningitis	44	1.9

High Income

Rank	Cause	Deaths (000s)	%
1	Congenital anomalies	19	20.5
2	Prematurity and low birth weight	17	17.6
3	Neonatal infections[a]	14	15.0
4	Birth asphyxia and birth trauma	7	7.7
5	Road traffic accidents	4	4.1
6	Lower respiratory infections	3	3.6
7	Endocrine disorders	3	2.8
8	Diarrhoeal diseases	3	2.7
9	Drownings	2	1.8
10	Violence	1	1.5

AIDS, acquired immunodeficiency syndrome; HIV, human immunodeficiency virus
[a]Includes severe neonatal infections and other non-infectious causes arising in the perinatal period.
Source: WHO (2004) (27)

Annex D

Table D3 Ages 10–19 years

World

Rank	Cause	Deaths (000s)	%
1	Road traffic accidents	136	9.6
2	Lower respiratory infections	111	7.8
3	Drownings	78	5.5
4	Self-inflicted injuries	71	5.0
5	Violence	60	4.3
6	Tuberculosis	57	4.0
7	HIV/AIDS	41	2.9
8	Meningitis	40	2.8
9	Malaria	35	2.4
10	Fires	33	2.4

Low Income

Rank	Cause	Deaths (000s)	%
1	Lower respiratory infections	93	10.5
2	Road traffic accidents	49	5.5
3	Tuberculosis	41	4.7
4	Self-inflicted injuries	40	4.5
5	HIV/AIDS	36	4.0
6	Meningitis	35	3.9
7	Drownings	32	3.6
8	Malaria	32	3.6
9	Fires	28	3.2
10	Violence	22	2.5

Middle Income

Rank	Cause	Deaths (000s)	%
1	Road traffic accident	74	15.1
2	Drownings	45	9.0
3	Homicide	35	7.1
4	Self-inflicted injuries	27	5.5
5	Lower respiratory infections	18	3.6
6	Leukaemia	17	3.5
7	Tuberculosis	15	3.1
8	Congenital anomalies	9	1.8
9	Falls	8	1.7
10	Epilepsy	8	1.6

High Income

Rank	Cause	Deaths (000s)	%
1	Road traffic accidents	13	31.7
2	Self-inflicted injuries	5	11.2
3	Violence	3	7.2
4	Leukaemia	1	3.4
5	Drownings	1	3.3
6	Congenital anomalies	1	3.1
7	Poisonings	1	2.4
8	Endocrine disorders	1	2.2
9	Falls	1	1.2
10	Lower respiratory infections	0	1.1

AIDS, acquired immunodeficiency syndrome; HIV, human immunodeficiency virus
Source: WHO (2004) (27)

Table D4 Ages 20–59 years

World

Rank	Cause	Deaths (000s)	%
1	HIV/AIDS	1668	10.6
2	Ischaemic heart disease	1405	8.9
3	Tuberculosis	936	5.9
4	Cerebrovascular disease	857	5.4
5	Road traffic accidents	808	5.1
6	Self-inflicted injuries	574	3.6
7	Lower respiratory infections	483	3.1
8	Violence	462	2.9
9	Cirrhosis of the liver	384	2.4
10	Chronic obstructive pulmonary disease	369	2.3

Low Income

Rank	Cause	Deaths (000s)	%
1	HIV	1157	15.4
2	Ischaemic heart disease	637	8.5
3	Tuberculosis	615	8.2
4	Maternal conditions	378	5.0
5	Lower respiratory infections	318	4.2
6	Cerebrovascular disease	293	3.9
7	Road traffic accidents	281	3.7
8	Chronic obstructive pulmonary disease	219	2.9
9	Self-inflicted injuries	217	2.9
10	Violence	186	2.5

Middle Income

Rank	Cause	Deaths (000s)	%
1	Ischaemic heart disease	630	8.9
2	Cerebrovascular disease	512	7.3
3	HIV/AIDS	491	7.0
4	Road traffic accidents	456	6.5
5	Tuberculosis	318	4.5
6	Self-inflicted injuries	264	3.7
7	Violence	255	3.6
8	Cirrhosis of the liver	211	3.0
9	Trachea, bronchus and lung cancers	203	2.9
10	Stomach cancer	168	2.4

High Income

Rank	Cause	Deaths (000s)	%
1	Ischaemic heart disease	138	11.1
2	Self-inflicted injuries	93	7.5
3	Trachea, bronchus and lung cancers	85	6.9
4	Road traffic accidents	70	5.6
5	Cirrhosis of the liver	53	4.3
6	Cerebrovascular disease	52	4.2
7	Breast cancer	49	4.0
8	Colon and rectum cancers	39	3.1
9	Diabetes mellitus	28	2.3
10	Poisonings	27	2.2

AIDS, acquired immunodeficiency syndrome; HIV, human immunodeficiency virus
Source: WHO (2004) (27)

Annex D

Table D5 Ages 60+ years

World

Rank	Cause	Deaths (000s)	%
1	Ischaemic heart disease	5770	**19.1**
2	Cerebrovascular disease	4822	**16.0**
3	Chronic obstructive pulmonary disease	2651	**8.8**
4	Lower respiratory infections	1623	**5.4**
5	Trachea, bronchus and lung cancers	990	**3.3**
6	Diabetes mellitus	863	**2.9**
7	Hypertensive disease	805	**2.7**
8	Stomach cancer	572	**1.9**
9	Colon and rectum cancers	491	**1.6**
10	Nephritis and nephrosis	478	**1.6**

Low Income

Rank	Cause	Deaths (000s)	%
1	Ischaemic heart disease	1780	**20.8**
2	Cerebrovascular disease	1149	**13.4**
3	Lower respiratory infections	830	**9.7**
4	Chronic obstructive pulmonary disease	712	**8.3**
5	Diabetes mellitus	264	**3.1**
6	Tuberculosis	194	**2.3**
7	Nephritis and nephrosis	160	**1.9**
8	Hypertensive disease	156	**1.8**
9	Diarrhoeal diseases	138	**1.6**
10	Mouth and oropharynx cancers	115	**1.3**

Middle Income

Rank	Cause	Deaths (000s)	%
1	Cerebrovascular disease	2948	**20.0**
2	Ischaemic heart disease	2762	**18.7**
3	Chronic obstructive pulmonary disease	1665	**11.3**
4	Hypertensive disease	516	**3.5**
5	Lower respiratory infections	501	**3.4**
6	Trachea, bronchus and lung cancers	486	**3.3**
7	Diabetes mellitus	399	**2.7**
8	Stomach cancer	378	**2.6**
9	Liver cancer	236	**1.6**
10	Oesophagus cancer	222	**1.5**

High Income

Rank	Cause	Deaths (000s)	%
1	Ischaemic heart disease	1227	**17.8**
2	Cerebrovascular disease	725	**10.5**
3	Trachea, bronchus and lung cancers	399	**5.8**
4	Lower respiratory infections	293	**4.2**
5	Alzheimer and other dementias	276	**4.0**
6	Chronic obstructive pulmonary disease	275	**4.0**
7	Colon and rectum cancers	232	**3.4**
8	Diabete mellitus	200	**2.9**
9	Hypertensive disease	132	**1.9**
10	Stomach cancer	123	**1.8**

AIDS, acquired immunodeficiency syndrome; HIV, human immunodeficiency virus
Source: WHO (2004) (*27*)

Glossary

Age-standardized rate	A rate designed to minimize the effects of differences in age composition when comparing rates for different populations.
ACME	Automated Classification of Medical Entities; this program automates the underlying cause-of-death coding rules. The input to ACME is the multiple cause-of-death codes (from the ICD) assigned to each entity (e.g. disease condition, accident or injury) listed on cause-of-death certifications, preserving the location and order as reported by the certifier. ACME then applies the WHO rules to the ICD codes and selects an underlying cause of death. ACME has become the de facto international standard for the automated selection of the underlying cause of death.
Birth	See "Live birth".
Capture–recapture	Capture–recapture methods can be used to assess the completeness of registration. The basic idea is to use two separate sources or methods to identify births or deaths, and to examine the proportion of cases identified by the second method that were also identified by the first. From this information, it is possible (through mathematical models) to estimate the total number of cases.
	Capture–recapture can be used to assist in monitoring trends over time, but it assumes closed populations.
Causes of death	"All those diseases, morbid conditions or injuries that either resulted in or contributed to death and the circumstances of the accident or violence that produced any such injuries." (27)
Census	See "Population census".
Certification of cause of death	Process by which a doctor confirms the fact of death, states the causes leading to it and issues a certificate that specifies the underlying cause of death, according to the rules and procedures of the ICD.
Child mortality	Deaths of children under 5 years of age (i.e. in the exact age range 0–4 years old); usually measured as the probability of a neonate dying before their 5th birthday.
Citizen	A person who holds the legal nationality of the country they are living in and, as such, benefits from all the constitutional rights of that country but also is subject to the obligations and regulations that apply to its citizens.
Civil registration	"The continuous, permanent, compulsory, and universal recording of the occurrence and characteristics of vital events (live births, deaths, fetal deaths, marriages and divorces) and other civil status events pertaining to the population as provided by decree, law or regulation, in accordance with the legal requirements in each country. Civil registration establishes and provides legal documentation of such events. These records are also the best source of vital statistics" (1).
Civil registrar	Official charged with the responsibility for registering vital events in a defined area (e.g. a country, district, municipality or parish) and for reporting these for legal and statistical purposes.
Civil society	The voluntary participation of citizens in the civic and social bodies that form the basis of a functioning society, as opposed to state and commercial institutions.
Completeness of registration	The extent to which all births or deaths are registered in a population; usually expressed as a percentage of the total deaths and births in a population. Sometimes also referred to as the coverage of registration. Any deviation from complete coverage is measured by coverage error.
Delayed registration	The registration of a vital event after the prescribed period specified in existing laws, rules or regulations (including any specified grace period). Delayed registration is usually considered to be the registration of a vital event one year or more after the event has occurred. (Not to be confused with "late registration".)
Demographic surveillance	The practice of registering, on a continuous basis, all demographic events (including cause of death, which is usually assessed by verbal autopsy) in one or more geographically defined populations. The major drawback of demographic surveillance is that it does not produce nationally representative data but only information for the specific sites chosen.
Fetal death	"Death prior to the complete expulsion or extraction from its mother of a product of conception, irrespective of the duration of the pregnancy; the death is indicated by the fact that after such separation the fetus does not breathe or show any evidence of life, such as beating of the heart, pulsation of the umbilical cord, or definite movement of voluntary muscles" (27).

Glossary

Household surveys	Household surveys are generally unreliable sources of data on adult and cause-specific mortality, because of the relative rarity of such deaths and the limitations of sample size. Due to sample-size limitations, reliable estimates are usually only possible at national level and for major subregions. Population-based surveys include more detailed questions on mortality and fertility than can be asked during a census, and can thus be used to generate estimates of fertility, child and adult mortality. DHS, PAPCHILD and MICS are examples of survey programmes that have yielded useful estimates of vital statistics rates, particularly fertility and child mortality.
ICD-10	International statistical classification of diseases and related health problems, 10th revision (ICD-10; sometimes shortened to the International classification of diseases) (28). ICD-10 is a classification maintained by the WHO for coding diseases, signs, symptoms and other factors causing morbidity and mortality. It is used worldwide for classifying morbidity and mortality statistics, and is designed to promote international comparability in the collection, processing, classification and presentation of statistics.
Ill-defined cause of death	A collection of vague diagnoses that should not be used as the underlying cause of death, and consisting of: "symptoms, signs and abnormal clinical and laboratory findings, not elsewhere classified" (Chapter XIII of ICD-10). For further information, see Section 4.1.10 in ICD-10, Volume 2.
Infant mortality	Deaths in children occurring before their first birthday, usually measured as infant deaths per 1000 live births.
Late registration	Registration of a vital event after the prescribed time period but within a specified grace period. Since the grace period is usually considered to be one year following the vital event, late registration means the registration of a vital event within one year of the event occurring. (Not to be confused with delayed registration.)
Life expectancy	Average number of years a person could expect to live if current mortality trends continue for the rest of that person's life.
Life table	A tabular display of life expectancies and the probability of dying at each age (or age group) for a given population, calculated from age-specific death rates prevailing at that time. The life table gives a complete picture of a population's mortality.
Live birth	The result of the complete expulsion or extraction from its mother of a product of conception, irrespective of the duration of pregnancy, which after such separation breathes or shows any other evidence of life, such as beating of the heart, pulsation of the umbilical cord or definite movement of voluntary muscles, whether or not the umbilical cord has been cut or the placenta is attached; each product of such a birth is considered to be live born.
Maternal death	Death of a woman while pregnant or within 42 days of termination of pregnancy (irrespective of the duration and the site of the pregnancy) from any cause related to or aggravated by the pregnancy or its management, but not from accidental or incidental causes.
Metadata	Information about data including definitions, attributes (e.g. name, size and data type), sources, estimation methods and other characteristics.
Millennium Development Goals (MDGs)	Eight major development goals and associated targets and indicators, endorsed by Member States of the UN in the year 2000.
Mode of death	The way a person died; for example, "respiratory failure". To write this on a death certificate is not sufficient because it does not indicate what disease or condition caused the death.
Mortality rate	The ratio of the number of people dying in a year to the total mid-year population in which the deaths occurred. This rate is also called the crude death rate. The mortality rate may be standardized when comparing mortality rates over time (or between countries), to take account of differences in the population; the rate is then called the age-standardized death rate.
Notification	The paper documentation needed to obtain a permit to bury a deceased person, and that serves as documentary evidence for the civil registration to register the birth or death.
Perinatal mortality	Deaths occurring in the perinatal period that commences at 22 completed weeks (154 days) of gestation (the time when birth weight is normally 500 g) and ends 7 completed days after birth (28).

Glossary

Population census	The total process of collecting, compiling, evaluating, analysing and publishing or otherwise disseminating demographic, economic and social data pertaining, at a specified time, to all persons in a country or in a well delimited part of a country (*35*). Data from population censuses can be used to estimate birth and death rates. Also, they can provide the best source of data on at-risk populations (numerators and denominators) in small geographical or administrative areas, and the baseline for sample vital registration.
Population register	A mechanism for the continuous recording of selected information pertaining to each member of the resident population of a country or area, making it possible to have up-to-date information about the size and characteristics of the population at selected points in time. Because of the nature of a population register, both its organization and operation should have a legal basis. Population registers start with a base consisting of an inventory of the inhabitants of an area and their characteristics (e.g. date of birth, sex, marital status, place of birth, place of residence, citizenship and language). To assist in locating a record for a particular person, household or family in a population register, a unique identification number is provided for each entity.
	The population register can contain other socioeconomic data, such as occupation or education. The population register should be updated by births, deaths, marriages and divorces, which are part of the civil registration system of the country. The population register is also updated by migration. Thus, notifications of certain events, which may have been recorded originally in different administrative systems, are automatically linked to a population register on a current basis. The method and sources of updating should cover all changes, so that the characteristics of individuals in the register remain current (*1*).
Quality of data	In a vital statistics system, quality of data is usually measured according to the degree of completeness, accuracy, timeliness and availability.
Registrar general	The head of the civil registration office or department with jurisdiction usually extending over the entire national territory.
Registration	The formal act of reporting a birth or death, and obtaining a birth or death certificate issued by the civil registration authority.
Sample vital registration	The registration of all demographic events on a continuous basis (as in full civil registration) but only for a nationally representative sample of administrative areas for which a baseline population census has been taken. Cause of death is assessed from hospital records where these are available. In all other cases, death is first notified to the sample registration office, and the household is later visited and a verbal autopsy is conducted to determine the cause of death. The system yields nationally representative vital statistics that include the major causes of death. If properly conducted and carefully expanded, sample registration is the best way to gradually expand into a national civil registration system. However, if the population under surveillance is too small or not representative, the data will be biased or too small to yield reliable cause-specific death rates.
Sample vital registration with verbal autopsy (SAVVY)	The MEASURE Evaluation project based at the University of North Carolina at Chapel Hill and the United States Census Bureau have together created a series of sample vital registration with verbal autopsy (SAVVY) manuals for mortality surveillance.[10]
Stakeholders	Persons or institutions with a shared interest (financial or otherwise) in a given event, process or outcome.
Stillbirth	See "Fetal death".
Technical assistance	Development aid or cooperation provided by governmental and nongovernmental agencies to assist the economic, social and political development of populations. It also covers the transfer of knowledge from individual experts and scientists to countries as part of cooperative projects.
Underlying cause of death	Either (a) The disease or injury that initiated the train of morbid events leading directly to death; or (b) the circumstances of the accident or violence that produced the fatal injury. The underlying cause of death is used as the basis for the tabulation of mortality statistics.
Usual residence	The geographical location within a country, locality or other civil division where a specified person (the deceased, or a mother or father) usually resides. For vital statistics purposes, the place of usual residence for a birth or fetal death is the place where the mother usually resides.

---

[10] The manuals are available at http://www.cpc.unc.edu/measure/publications/index.php

Glossary

Verbal autopsy	A structured interview with caregivers or family members of households after a death occurs; used to determine the probable cause or causes of death in populations where most deaths occur outside health facilities, and where direct medical certification is rare.
Vital event	"The occurrence of a live birth, death, fetal death, marriage, divorce, adoption, legitimation, recognition of parenthood, annulment of marriage, or legal separation" (1).
Vital registration	All sanctioned modes of registering individuals and reporting on vital events.
Vital statistics	Statistics on vital events compiled from all sources of vital-events data (including civil registration, censuses and surveys).
Vital statistics system	"The total process of (a) collecting information by civil registration or enumeration on the frequency or occurrence of specified and defined vital events, as well as relevant characteristics of the events themselves and the person or persons concerned, and (b) compiling, processing, analyzing, evaluating, presenting, and disseminating these data in statistical form" (1).
WHO-FIC	WHO's Family of international disease and health related classifications.

References

1 United Nations (UN). *Principles and recommendations for a vital statistics system, Revision 2.* UN, 2001. http://unstats.un.org/unsd/publication/SeriesM/SeriesM_19rev2E.pdf

2 Health Metrics Network (HMN). *Framework and standards for country health information systems.* Geneva, World Health Organization, 2008. http://www.who.int/healthmetrics/documents/hmn_framework200803.pdf

3 Setel PW, Macfarlane SB, Szreter S et al. A scandal of invisibility: making everyone count by counting everyone. *Lancet,* 2007, 370(9598):1569–1577. http://www.ncbi.nlm.nih.gov/entrez/query.fcgi?cmd=Retrieve&db=PubMed&dopt=Citation&list_uids=18029007

4 Mahapatra P, Shibuya K, Lopez AD et al. Civil registration systems and vital statistics: successes and missed opportunities. *Lancet,* 2007, 370(9599):1653–1663. http://www.ncbi.nlm.nih.gov/entrez/query.fcgi?cmd=Retrieve&db=PubMed&dopt=Citation&list_uids=18029006

5 Lopez AD, AbouZahr C, Shibuya K et al. Keeping count: births, deaths, and causes of death. *Lancet,* 2007, 370(9601):1744–1746. http://www.ncbi.nlm.nih.gov/entrez/query.fcgi?cmd=Retrieve&db=PubMed&dopt=Citation&list_uids=18029004

6 Hill K, Lopez AD, Shibuya K et al. Interim measures for meeting needs for health sector data: births, deaths, and causes of death. *Lancet,* 2007. http://www.ncbi.nlm.nih.gov/entrez/query.fcgi?cmd=Retrieve&db=PubMed&dopt=Citation&list_uids=18029005

7 AbouZahr C, Cleland J, Coullare F et al. The way forward. *Lancet,* 2007, 370(9601):1791–1799. http://www.ncbi.nlm.nih.gov/entrez/query.fcgi?cmd=Retrieve&db=PubMed&dopt=Citation&list_uids=18029003

8 Health Metrics Network (HMN). *Monitoring vital events resource kit.* Geneva, World Health Organization, 2007. http://www.who.int/healthmetrics/tools/logbook/en/move/web/index.html

9 United Nations Children's Fund (UNICEF). Birth registration: rights from the start. *Innocenti Digest,* 2002.

10 Danel I, Bortman M. *An assessment of LAC's vital statistics system: the foundation of infant and materal mortality.* World Bank, 2008. http://siteresources.worldbank.org/HEALTHNUTRITIONANDPOPULATION/Resources/281627-1095698140167/LACVitalStat.pdf

11 Horton R. Counting for health. *Lancet,* 2007, 370(9598):1526–1526. http://www.ncbi.nlm.nih.gov/entrez/query.fcgi?cmd=Retrieve&db=PubMed&dopt=Citation&list_uids=18029008

12 Mathers CD, Fat DM, Inoue M et al. Counting the dead and what they died from: an assessment of the global status of cause of death data. *Bulletin of the World Health Organization,* 2005, 83(3):171–177. http://www.ncbi.nlm.nih.gov/entrez/query.fcgi?cmd=Retrieve&db=PubMed&dopt=Citation&list_uids=15798840

13 Health Metrics Network (HMN). *Guidance for the health information systems (HIS) strategic planning process* Geneva, World Health Organization, 2009.

14 Mahapatra P, Chalapati Rao PV. Cause of death reporting systems in India: a performance analysis. *National Medical Journal of India,* 2001, 14(3):154–162. http://www.ncbi.nlm.nih.gov/entrez/query.fcgi?cmd=Retrieve&db=PubMed&dopt=Citation&list_uids=11467144

15 Rao C, Bradshaw D, Mathers C. Improving death registration and statistics in developing countries: lessons from Sub-Saharan Africa *Southern African Journal of Demography,* 2004, 9(2):79–97.

16 Rao C, Lopez AD, Yang G et al. Evaluating national cause-of-death statistics: principles and application to the case of China. *Bulletin of the World Health Organization,* 2005, 83(8):618–625. http://www.ncbi.nlm.nih.gov/entrez/query.fcgi?cmd=Retrieve&db=PubMed&dopt=Citation&list_uids=16184281

17 Ruzicka LT, Lopez AD. The use of cause-of-death statistics for health situation assessment: national and international experiences. *World Health Statistics Quarterly,* 1990, 43(4):249–258. http://www.ncbi.nlm.nih.gov/entrez/query.fcgi?cmd=Retrieve&db=PubMed&dopt=Citation&list_uids=2293493

18 Pan American Health Organization/World Health Organization (PAHO/WHO). *Guide for the analysis of vital, morbidity, and health resources statistics – questionnaire 2.* PAHO, 2007.

19 United Nations (UN). *World population prospects: The 2008 revision population database.* New York, UN Department of Economic and Social Affairs Statistics Division, 2008. http://esa.un.org/unpp/

20 United Nations (UN). *Handbook on civil registration and vital statistics systems: management, operation and maintenance, No. 72.* UN Department of Economic and Social Affairs Statistics Division, 1998. http://unstats.un.org/unsd/pubs/gesgrid.asp?id=66

References

21. United Nations (UN). *Handbook on civil registration and vital statistics systems: preparation of a legal framework, No. 71.* UN Department of Economic and Social Affairs Statistics Division, 1998. http://unstats.un.org/unsd/pubs/gesgrid.asp?id=65

22. United Nations (UN). *Fundamental principles of official statistics.* New York, UN Statistics Division, 1994. http://unstats.un.org/unsd/dnss/gp/fundprinciples.aspx

23. Health Metrics Network (HMN). *Assessing the national health information system. an assessment tool – Version 4.* Geneva, World Health Organization, 2008.

24. World Health Organization (WHO). *Age standardization of rates: a new WHO standard.* Geneva, EIP/GPE/EBD, WHO, 2001. http://www.who.int/healthinfo/paper31.pdf

25. United Nations (UN). *Handbook on civil registration and vital statistics systems: policies and protocols for the release and archiving of individual records.* New York, UN Department of Economic and Social Affairs Statistics Division, 1998. http://unstats.un.org/unsd/publication/SeriesF/SeriesF_70E.pdf

26. Centres for Disease Control and Prevention (CDC). *Core curriculum for certifiers of underlying cause of death.* CDC, 2007. http://www.cdc.gov/nchs/data/icd9/CurriculumCertification03-08-078.pdf

27. World Health Organization (WHO). *International Classification of Diseases (ICD).* Geneva, WHO, 2004. http://www.who.int/classifications/icd/en/

28. World Health Organization (WHO). *International statistical classification of diseases and related health problems* Geneva, WHO, 2007. http://apps.who.int/classifications/apps/icd/icd10online/

29. Sibai AM. Mortality certification and cause-of-death reporting in developing countries. *Bulletin of the World Health Organization,* 2004, 82(2):83. http://www.ncbi.nlm.nih.gov/entrez/query.fcgi?cmd=Retrieve&db=PubMed&dopt=Citation&list_uids=15042227

30. Murray C, Lopez A. *Global health statistics.* Cambridge, MA, Harvard University Press, on behalf of the World Health Organization and the World Bank, 1996.

31. World Health Organization (WHO). *Verbal autopsy standards. Ascertaining and attributing cause of death.* Geneva, WHO, 2007. http://www.who.int/whosis/mort/verbalautopsystandards/en/index.html

32. World Health Organization (WHO). *Beyond the numbers: reviewing maternal deaths and complications to make pregnancy safer.* Geneva, WHO, 2004. http://www.who.int/making_pregnancy_safer/documents/9241591838/en/index.html

33. Becker R, Silvi J, Ma Fat D et al. A method for deriving leading causes of death. *Bulletin of the World Health Organization,* 2006, 84(4):297–304. http://www.ncbi.nlm.nih.gov/entrez/query.fcgi?cmd=Retrieve&db=PubMed&dopt=Citation&list_uids=16628303

34. Centers for Disease Control and Prevention (CDC). *Recommended framework for presenting injury mortality data.* 1997. ftp://ftp.cdc.gov/pub/Publications/mmwr/rr/rr4614.pdf

35. United Nations (UN). *Principles and recommendations for population and housing censuses, Revision 1.* UN 1997. http://unstats.un.org/unsd/pubs/gesgrid.asp?ID=127

WHO/IER/HSI/STM/2010.1

Rapid assessment of national civil registration and vital statistics systems

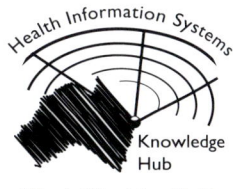
School of Population Health
University of Queensland

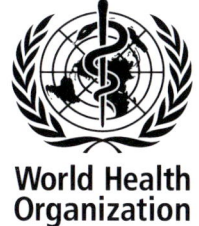
World Health Organization

Rapid assessment of national civil registration and vital statistics systems

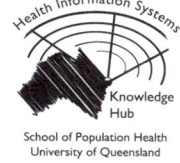
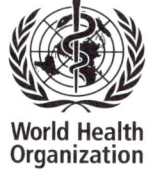

© World Health Organization 2010

All rights reserved. Publications of the World Health Organization can be obtained from WHO Press, World Health Organization, 20 Avenue Appia, 1211 Geneva 27, Switzerland (tel.: +41 22 791 3264; fax: +41 22 791 4857; e-mail: bookorders@who.int). Requests for permission to reproduce or translate WHO publications – whether for sale or for noncommercial distribution – should be addressed to WHO Press, at the above address (fax: +41 22 791 4806; e-mail: permissions@who.int).

The designations employed and the presentation of the material in this publication do not imply the expression of any opinion whatsoever on the part of the World Health Organization concerning the legal status of any country, territory, city or area or of its authorities, or concerning the delimitation of its frontiers or boundaries. Dotted lines on maps represent approximate border lines for which there may not yet be full agreement.

The mention of specific companies or of certain manufacturers' products does not imply that they are endorsed or recommended by the World Health Organization in preference to others of a similar nature that are not mentioned. Errors and omissions excepted, the names of proprietary products are distinguished by initial capital letters.

All reasonable precautions have been taken by the World Health Organization to verify the information contained in this publication. However, the published material is being distributed without warranty of any kind, either expressed or implied. The responsibility for the interpretation and use of the material lies with the reader. In no event shall the World Health Organization be liable for damages arising from its use.

Design by Robert Redding

Editing and production by Cadman Editing Services, Canberra

Printed in Malta by Progress Press Co. Ltd.

Acknowledgements

This assessment tool has been produced in parallel with the development of the World Health Organization (WHO) document *Improving the quality and use of birth, death and cause-of-death information*[1], which provides guidance for a standards-based review of country practices in civil registration and vital statistics. Lene Mikkelsen and Alan Lopez – from the School of Population Health, University of Queensland, Australia – co-wrote the original text. Valuable inputs to early drafts were provided by Vicki Bennett (School of Population Health, University of Queensland, Australia), Debbie Bradshaw (Medical Research Council, Cape Town, South Africa), John Cleland (London School of Hygiene and Tropical Medicine, London, United Kingdom), Francesca Grum (United Nations Statistics Division, New York, United States), Rafael Lozano (Institute for Health Metrics and Evaluation at the University of Washington, United States); Prasantha Mahapatra (Institute of Health Systems, Hyderabad, Andhra Pradesh, India), Cleone Rooney (Office of National Statistics, London, United Kingdom), Kenji Shibuya (University of Tokyo, Tokyo, Japan), Sue Walker (School of Public Health, Queensland University of Technology, Australia) and Eduardo Zacca (Ministry of Health, Havana, Cuba).

Particular thanks are due to the following country partners who tested the approach and provided valuable feedback: Estuardo Albán (Instituto Nacional de Estadistica y Censos, Ecuador), Lourdes J Hufana (National Statistical Office, Manila), Charity Tan (Department of Health, the Philippines) and Rasika Rampatige (Ministry of Health, Sri Lanka).

Important contributions were also provided by the following WHO staff: Mohamed Ali (WHO Eastern Mediterranean Region, Cairo, Egypt), Mark Amexo (Health Metrics Network, WHO, Geneva, Switzerland), Jun Gao (WHO Western Pacific Region, Manila, the Philippines), Alejandro Giusti (WHO Region of the Americas, Santiago, Chile), Fiona Gore (WHO, Geneva, Switzerland), Mie Inoue (WHO, Geneva, Switzerland), Robert Jakob (WHO, Geneva, Switzerland), Enrique Loyola (WHO European Region, Copenhagen, Denmark), Doris MaFat (WHO, Geneva, Switzerland), Fatima Marinho (WHO/Pan American Health Organization, Washington DC, USA), Lucille Nievera (WHO Country Office, Manila, the Philippines), Sunil Senanayake (WHO South-East Asia Region, Delhi, India) and William Soumbey-Alley (WHO African Region, Brazzaville, Congo).

Carla AbouZahr (WHO, Geneva, Switzerland) oversaw the development of the tool, with administrative assistance from Sue Piccolo and Petra Schuster. Financial support was provided by the Government of Japan, the Health Metrics Network, the WHO and the Health Information Systems Hub at the School of Population Health at the University of Queensland, Australia.

Acronyms

AIDS	acquired immunodeficiency virus
HIV	human immunodeficiency virus
ICD-10	International statistical classification of diseases and related health problems, 10th revision
WHO	World Health Organization

---

[1] *Improving the quality and use of birth, death and cause-of-death information: guidance for a standards-based review of country practices.* Geneva, World Health Organization, 2010.

Contents

Acknowledgements	iii
Acronyms	iii
Background and rationale	1
The rapid assessment tool and its application	2
Rapid assessment questions	4
Legal framework for civil registration and vital statistics	4
Registration infrastructure and resources	5
Organization and functioning of the vital statistics system	6
Completeness of registration of births and deaths	7
Data storage and transmission	8
ICD-compliant practices and certification within and outside hospitals	9
Practices affecting the quality of cause-of-death data	10
ICD coding practices	10
Coder qualification and training, and quality of coding	11
Data quality and plausibility checks	12
Data access, dissemination and use	13

Background and rationale

In most countries, statistics on births, deaths, marriages, divorces and fetal deaths are recorded through the government's civil registration system, which creates a permanent record of each event. The records derived from civil registration systems have two main uses. First, they are personal legal documents, required by citizens as proof of facts (e.g. age, identity) surrounding events. These records are used, for example, to establish family relationships and inheritance rights, provide proof of age and establish rights based on age (e.g. school entry, driving privileges), provide proof of marriage or divorce and the right to marry, and provide evidence of death. Second, the data derived from these records form the basis of a country's vital statistics system.

Vital statistics are used to derive the fundamental demographic and epidemiological measures that are needed in national planning across multiple sectors such as education, labour and health. They are also critical for a wide range of government activities (e.g. population registers and other administrative registers) and commercial enterprises (e.g. life insurance, marketing of products). In the health sector, vital statistics form the core of a country's health information system; they:

- permit understanding of the prevalence and distribution of mortality due to diseases and injury, identification of health inequalities and priorities, monitoring of trends, and evaluation of the impact and effectiveness of health programmes;

- provide (when timely and complete) a reliable way to measure baseline levels and monitor progress towards global goals such as the Millennium Development Goals, and are important in understanding emerging health challenges due to, for example, noncommunicable diseases, injuries and human immunodeficiency virus/acquired immunodeficiency syndrome (HIV/AIDS);

- enable tracking of national processes such as health sector reform, poverty reduction strategies and development efforts overall; and

- support planning, monitoring and evaluation in decentralized health systems[1], by providing information on health conditions at a local level.

Civil registration records are the best source of vital statistics. However, such systems are often weak or incomplete in developing countries. In countries where the civil registration system lacks complete coverage, or has major deficiencies due to issues of quality and timeliness, it may be necessary, on an interim basis, to use alternative sources to generate vital statistics. Sources for such interim data include population censuses, household sample surveys, demographic surveillance in sentinel sites and sample registration systems. Although these sources can and do generate measures of vital events, they do not provide individuals with the legal benefits of civil registration systems.

The World Health Organization (WHO), working with the University of Queensland in Australia, developed a comprehensive guide to support countries who wish to improve their civil registration and vital statistics systems. During the guide's development and field-testing phase, countries suggested that, before undertaking the detailed review, it would be useful to first carry out a rapid assessment to quickly evaluate the strengths and weaknesses of the current system. The results of this rapid assessment could then be used to make the case for a more detailed assessment.

This rapid assessment tool has therefore been developed to accompany the comprehensive guide, and countries are advised to apply it before undertaking a full review of their systems. It is available as both text and a spreadsheet, for ease of compilation of data. Both tools have been extensively peer reviewed by technical experts, and field tested in three countries.

---

[1] *Improving the quality and use of birth, death and cause-of-death information: Guidance for a standards-based review of country practices.* Geneva, World Health Organization, 2010.

The rapid assessment tool and its application

The rapid assessment tool consists of 25 questions about how the civil registration and vital statistics systems function (see "Rapid assessment questions", below). The questions are grouped into 11 areas:

- legal framework for civil registration and vital statistics;
- registration infrastructure and resources;
- organization and functioning of the vital statistics system;
- completeness of birth and death registration;
- data storage and transmission;
- *International statistical classification of diseases and related health problems* (ICD)[2]-compliant practices and certification within and outside hospitals;
- practices affecting the quality of cause-of-death data;
- ICD coding practices;
- coder qualification and training, and quality of coding;
- data quality and plausibility checks; and
- data access, dissemination and use.

Each question allows countries to select one of four scenarios (labelled A–D) describing a typical range of hypothetical situations. A numeric value (from 3 to 0) is attached to each scenario, allowing a total score to be obtained. The score has no scientific value and should only be taken as a rough indication of the functionality and quality of the civil registration and vital statistics systems. Some countries might find that the score can be used to help decide whether there is a need to carry out the comprehensive review. The rapid assessment tool is not a *replacement* for the detailed procedures described in the comprehensive guide; instead, it provides a quick overview of how well or how poorly a country's overall system is functioning.

Rather than the scores themselves, it is the process used to arrive at the scores that is important. The rapid assessment is *not a questionnaire* that one person should attempt to find suitable replies to; rather, it is a *group exercise* and should therefore be undertaken by a group of individuals knowledgeable in civil registration and vital statistics. The questions in the tool are designed to incite a discussion among senior staff responsible for various aspects of the civil registration and vital statistics systems. The composition of the team completing the assessment will vary by country, but it should include staff from national agencies involved with the collection or production of vital statistics such as the national statistics office, ministry of health and office of the registrar general. In principle, this same group would lead and oversee the comprehensive assessment completed using the detailed assessment tool.

The rapid assessment can be carried out in different ways. The group can meet and discuss each question before reaching a consensus on the overall country score. Alternatively, individual group members can score each question after the group discussion and the scores can then be averaged to produce a final result. Based on pilot experiences, the time needed for discussion of the issues raised by the questions would be around two hours.

Table 1 shows how the letter denoting a particular scenario for a question relates to the score.

Table 1 Scoring of scenarios for rapid assessment

Scenario	A	B	C	D
Score	3	2	1	0

The group should discuss and score all questions. If a particular scenario does not precisely define the situation in a country, the scenario most closely describing current practice is selected. A comments section is provided

---

[2] *International statistical classification of diseases and related health problems.* 10th Revision, version for 2007. Available at: http://apps.who.int/classifications/apps/icd/icd10online/

to enable respondents to provide additional detail or points of clarification for future reference. Total numeric scores are then converted into percentages. The spreadsheet version of the assessment questions will automatically calculate the scores and convert the absolute numbers into a percentage score. The spreadsheet tool can be downloaded from http://www.who.int/healthinfo/en/.

Based on the score obtained, the functioning of the national system can be situated.

Table 2 shows the ratings for the range of possible scores, and outlines the action required for each rating.

It is clear from Table 2 that countries with ratings below 65% will have much to gain from the careful application of the comprehensive WHO guide, and that even in countries with a score of 65–84%, the comprehensive review will be useful in identifying specific weaknesses.

A central tenet of the assessment approach is that the rapid assessment should be completed through a process of discussion among all group members leading to a common view on the issue. Thus, the purpose of the assessment is not simply to answer a question and decide on a score, but rather to engage in discussion on the possible weaknesses and strengths of the system, which will then be explored more fully in applying the full WHO guide, where necessary.

In some countries, the civil registration system is not the main vehicle for generating certain vital statistics, especially causes of death. Other mechanisms used include sample registration systems (e.g. India), disease surveillance points (e.g. China) and data collection through ministries of health (e.g. many countries in Latin America and the Caribbean). In such settings, it is important to distinguish between statistics derived from the civil registration system and those derived from alternative sources. This should be noted in the comments section of the questionnaire, because the rapid assessment is based on the premise that civil registration systems are the best source of vital statistics.

Table 2 Scores, ratings and actions required for rapid assessment

Score (%)	Rating	Actions required
<34	Dysfunctional	System requires substantial improvement in all areas
35–64	Weak	Many aspects of the system do not function well, and multiple issues require attention
65–84	Functional but inadequate	System works but some elements function poorly and require attention; specific weaknesses of the system should be identified by completing the comprehensive review
85–100	Satisfactory	Minor adjustments may be required in an otherwise well-functioning system

Rapid assessment questions
Legal framework for civil registration and vital statistics

1. Does the country have legislation that states that birth and death registration is compulsory?

Option	Response
A	Yes – the country has adequate and enforced legislation on civil registration, stating that registration of births and deaths is compulsory
B	Yes – the country has legislation on civil registration stating that registration of births and deaths is compulsory but it is in need of amendments
C	Yes – legislation exists but it is not enforced
D	No – there is no law that makes it obligatory to register births and deaths

Comments:
_____
_____

2. Does the country have regulations that oblige all medical establishments to report all vital events to the vital statistics system within a given time?

Option	Response
A	Yes – all medical establishments (public, private, social insurance, others) report these events to the vital statistics system in a timely manner
B	Yes – regulations exist but not all medical establishments report the events
C	No - regulations only cover public medical establishments
D	No – no regulations exist

Comments:
_____
_____

3. Does the country have legislation that states that death has to be certified by cause, and specifies who can certify the cause of death?

Option	Response
A	Yes – cause of death must be indicated on the death certificate according to International statistical classification of diseases and related health problems (ICD) rules and procedures, and can only be certified by a medical doctor
B	Cause of death must be indicated on the death certificate but it is not specified who can certify the cause
C	Cause of death must be indicated but only broad categories of cause are necessary, and the (non-medical) registrar or another local official is usually the certifier
D	No – it is not necessary to indicate the cause of death on the death certificate or at any stage of the registration of death

Comments:
_____
_____

Registration infrastructure and resources

4. Are there adequate numbers of civil registration offices or registration points to cover the whole country?

Option	Response
A	Yes – the country has sufficient places where citizens can register births and deaths
B	Urban areas are well covered but there is only partial coverage of rural areas
C	Only the urban areas are well covered
D	No – only the capital city has registration offices

Comments:
_____
_____

5. Do civil registration offices have adequate equipment to carry out their functions (for example, forms, telephones, photocopiers and computers)?

Option	Response
A	Yes – necessary supplies such as forms, paper and pens are adequate, and equipment such as telephones, photocopiers, and computers is widely available
B	Supplies such as forms, paper and pens are generally available everywhere, but there are widespread shortages of telephones, photocopiers and computers
C	In peripheral offices, supplies are often short, and only the central or provincial offices have telephones, photocopiers and computers
D	No – availability of both supplies and equipment is a problem in all civil registration offices

Comments:
_____
_____

6. Have registrars received training to carry out their functions?

Option	Response
A	Yes – all registrars have received adequate training
B	All registrars receive some training but the training is insufficient, and skills and knowledge are largely acquired on the job
C	Most registrars (particularly in smaller offices) receive only on-the-job training
D	No – lack of training is a serious problem and has a negative effect on the functioning of civil registration

Comments:
_____
_____

Organization and functioning of the vital statistics system

7. How well do the different government agencies and departments responsible for civil registration and vital statistics systems collaborate? (These include departments of health, civil registration and local government, statistics, and others)

Option	Response
A	The involved agencies collaborate very well and there is an interagency committee to ensure that the civil registration and vital statistics systems interact seamlessly
B	Although there is no formal interagency committee, the agencies involved have regular meetings to identify and resolve problems
C	There is no interagency committee, which delays efforts to resolve problems and can lead to serious data quality issues and bottlenecks (e.g. in data transfer)
D	There is little interagency collaboration, with the various agencies functioning independently, resulting in problems such as duplication of work and inconsistencies in the estimates derived from vital statistics issued by each agency

Comments:
_____
_____

8. Can the vital statistics system generate both national and subnational statistics on births and deaths each year?

Option	Response
A	Yes – annual statistics are generated on births, deaths, and causes of death by sex and age at both national and for all subnational levels
B	Annual statistics on births and deaths by sex and age are generated at national and subnational levels, but statistics on cause of death by sex and age are only available nationally
C	The vital statistics system can only generate births and deaths by sex and age for reporting regions and not for the whole country; cause of death data are obtained only from hospitals
D	No – the information collected by the civil registration system is not compiled for statistical purposes

Comments:
_____
_____

Completeness of registration of births and deaths

Before replying to questions 9 and 10, carefully read Box 1, which explains the concept of completeness. If no recent completeness estimates exist for birth and death registrations, they can be calculated using the simple method indicated in Box 1.

9. According to the most recent evaluation, how complete is birth registration in your country?

Option	Response
A	A recent evaluation (that is, in the last 10 years) showed that completeness of birth registration was 90% or higher (specify the date and method used to calculate completeness, and who calculated it)
B	A recent evaluation showed that completeness of birth registration was between 70% and 89% (specify the date and method used to calculate completeness, and who calculated it)
C	A recent evaluation showed that completeness of birth registration was between 50% and 69% (specify the date and method used to calculate completeness, and who calculated it)
D	*Either* – a recent evaluation showed that less than 50% of all births were registered (specify the date and method used to calculate completeness, and who calculated it) *or* – there has not been a recent evaluation of the completeness of birth registration

Comments - include date, method used, institution/person who calculated the completeness level:

_____

_____

10. According to the most recent evaluation, how complete is death registration in your country?

Option	Response
A	A recent evaluation (that is, in the last 10 years) showed that completeness of death registration was 90% or higher (specify the date and method used to calculate completeness, and who calculated it)
B	A recent evaluation showed that completeness of death registration was between 70% and 89% (specify the date and method used to calculate completeness, and who calculated it)
C	A recent evaluation showed that completeness of death registration was between 50% and 69% (specify the date and method used to calculate completeness, and who calculated it)
D	*Either* – a recent evaluation showed that less than 50% of all deaths were registered (specify the date and method used to calculate completeness and who calculated it) *or* – there has not been a recent evaluation of the completeness of death registration

Comments - include date, method used, institution/person who calculated the completeness level:

_____

Data storage and transmission

11. How are birth and death records transmitted from local and regional offices to a central storage in the capital city?

Option	Response
A	All information is exchanged electronically from local to regional offices, then to a central office
B	Paper copies are sent from local offices to the regional office and processed there for electronic transmission to the central office
C	The system is still mainly paper based, with copies sent from local offices to the regional office, where they are scanned, then sent to the central office for processing
D	Paper copies are used throughout the system to transfer birth and death records to a central storage facility

Comments:
_____
_____

12. What procedures are in place to ensure that all local and regional offices report to the central office within agreed times?

Option	Response
A	There is an agreed schedule for reporting to the central office, with reporting deadlines taken seriously and closely monitored – it is rarely necessary to send out reminders
B	An agreed schedule for reporting to the central office exists and this is largely adhered to – delays in local and regional offices are usually communicated to the central office
C	Although there is a schedule of reporting from local and regional offices, this is not strictly adhered to and there is currently little that the central office can do to ensure the timely transfer of data
D	The local and regional offices report to the central office with erratic timelines, and there is little effort by the central office to encourage more timely and regular reporting

Comments:
_____
_____

ICD-compliant practices and certification within and outside hospitals

13. Does the country use the standard International form of medical certificate of cause of death for reporting?

Option	Response
A	Yes – the form is always used by doctors to certify cause of death
B	The form is always used when deaths occur in health facilities, but is not generally used outside health facilities
C	The form is used to certify death only in major hospitals
D	No – the form is not used for certifying causes of death

Comments:
_____
_____

14. When medical certification of cause of death is rare, is verbal autopsy[1] routinely used to determine the cause of death? (This question does not apply to countries where all deaths generally are medically certified as part of civil registration. Countries in this category should give themselves a score of 3)

Option	Response
A	Yes – verbal autopsy is routinely applied to certify death using the international standard tool[2] or a similar questionnaire based on this
B	Verbal autopsy using the international standard tool is progressively being introduced but is not currently in general use
C	Verbal autopsy is used but is not based on the international standard tool
D	Verbal autopsy is not routinely used to determine cause of death in cases where the death is not certified by a physician

Comments:
_____
_____

---

[1] A verbal autopsy is a structured interview with caregivers or family members of households after a death occurs that is used to determine the probable cause or causes of death in populations where most deaths occur outside health facilities, and where direct medical certification is rare.

[2] *Verbal autopsy standards: ascertaining and attributing cause of death.* Geneva, World Health Organization, 2007.

Practices affecting the quality of cause-of-death data

15. What training do doctors receive for certifying the cause of death?

Option	Response
A	All medical students are introduced to the ICD during their studies, and are taught how to certify cause of death and correctly complete the medical death certificate
B	No special training in the ICD or death certification is included in the medical curriculum, but all medical students learn about the ICD and death certification during their internships
C	No special training in the ICD or death certification is included in the medical curriculum, and only limited on-the-job training is available during internships
D	No training or on-the-job instructions in the ICD and death certification is given to doctors

Comments:
_____
_____

16. What percentage of causes of death in your country are classified as "Ill-defined and unknown causes of mortality" (as defined in Chapter XVIII of ICD-10[1])?

Option	Response
A	<10%
B	10–19%
C	20–39%
D	40% or more

Comments:
_____
_____

ICD coding practices

17. In your country, is cause of death coded according to a national language version of the ICD?

Option	Response
A	Yes – ICD coding is done using a national language version of the ICD or a nationally agreed international language
B	ICD coding is done, but no national language version of the ICD is available, which makes the coders' task more difficult
C	ICD coding is done according to a short list in the national language
D	No – the ICD is not used

Comments:
_____
_____

---

[1] *International statistical classification of diseases and related health problems.* 10th Revision, version for 2007. Available at: http://apps.who.int/classifications/apps/icd/icd10online/

Coder qualification and training, and quality of coding

18. What qualifications do mortality coders have for coding mortality in accordance with ICD principles and rules?

Option	Response
A	Mortality coders must pass a formal test following a compulsory and intensive ICD-training course; additional courses are offered as needed
B	Mortality coders are given a short training course in the ICD and pass a basic test. Complex issues are learnt on the job from more experienced coders
C	New coders are instructed by more experienced coders; new coders are given the ICD volumes and expected to learn on the job
D	New coders are provided with minimal instructions from other coders and receive incomplete ICD materials

Comments:
_____
_____

19. What quality assurance procedures are in place for checking the coding?

Option	Response
A	A national regulatory procedure is in place to periodically review the quality of coded certificates, and feedback is given to coders so they can improve if necessary
B	National evaluation of a random sample of coded certificates takes place occasionally to monitor the quality of the coding
C	Quality evaluation is left to local supervisors who check the work of individual coders on an ad hoc basis
D	No procedures exist and no evaluations of the quality of coding have been carried out

Comments:
_____
_____

Data quality and plausibility checks

20. What consistency and plausibility checks on fertility and mortality levels are carried out before the data are released?

Option	Response
A	Checks on overall levels of fertility and mortality derived from the vital statistics data are made routinely by calculating rates and comparing these over time; rates are also compared to data derived from other sources, such as censuses and surveys
B	Checks on overall levels of fertility and mortality derived from vital statistics data are undertaken by calculating rates and comparing these to earlier time series
C	Checks are limited to computer programmes that simply look for compilation errors before the data are published
D	No specific checks are routinely carried out for data quality and plausibility of birth and death statistics

Comments:
_____
_____

21. What consistency and plausibility checks are applied to data on cause of death?

Option	Response
A	In addition to checking the stability of patterns in cause of death over time, the proportion of ill-defined and unknown deaths is routinely monitored, and the age and sex patterns for major causes of death are checked for plausibility
B	Routine checks of the consistency of patterns in cause of death are made to ensure that mortality from any disease group does not vary significantly from year to year, and that any fluctuations can be explained
C	Checks are limited to automated checks for compilation and data entry errors
D	There are no consistency and plausibility checks routinely carried out on data for cause of death

Comments:
_____
_____

Data access, dissemination and use

22. Does the country publish or make available annual numbers of births disaggregated by sex, age and geographical or administrative region?

Option	Response
A	Yes - annual data on births are published by all three disaggregations (sex, age and geographical or administrative region) Please indicate name of publication or web address where these data can be found
B	Annual data on births are published according to any two disaggregations
C	Annual data on births are available but disaggregated by sex only
D	No annual statistics on birth are published

Comments:
_____
_____

23. Does the country publish or make available annual numbers of deaths disaggregated by sex, age and geographical or administrative region?

Option	Response
A	Yes - annual data on deaths are published by all three disaggregations (sex, age and geographical or administrative region). Please indicate name of publication or web address where these data can be found
B	Annual data on deaths are published according to any two of the above disaggregations
C	Annual data on deaths are available but disaggregated by sex only
D	No annual statistics on death are published

Comments:
_____
_____

24. **What is the delay between the reference year and the time when detailed national statistics on cause of death, classified by sex and age, are made available to the public?**

Option	Response
A	Less than 2 years
B	More than 2 years but less than 3 years
C	More than 3 years but less than 5 years
D	5 years or more

Comments:
_____
_____

25. **How are data on vital events used for policy and programme purposes? (The group should discuss actual examples of where vital registration data are used)**

Option	Response
A	Data on births, deaths, and causes of death are widely used for socioeconomic planning and for monitoring the health status of the population, including the use of data on cause of death for public health purposes
B	Data on births and deaths are used for reporting on health-related indicators such as the Millennium Development Goals and other national health-related goals, but cause-specific data are rarely used for public health purposes
C	Only data on births are used for reporting on some indicators, such as fertility
D	Data from the civil registration and vital statistics systems are not routinely used for policy and programme purposes

Comments:
_____
_____

Box 1
Calculation of completeness of vital statistics

Completeness is a measure of the extent to which the births and deaths that occur in a country in a given year are registered by the civil registration system. There are various demographic techniques for estimating the completeness of deaths registration, such as the Bennett–Horiuchi, Chanrasekaran–Deming, and Brass Growth Balance methods.[1] Alternatively, it is possible to estimate completeness by dividing the actual number of registered births (or deaths) in the country by the total estimated number of births (or deaths) in the country for the same period, and multiplying by 100. A simple way to measure completeness in this way is to use an independent estimate of the number of births (or deaths) in the country. If no reliable national estimate is available, then an international estimate can be used. For example, each year the United Nations estimates birth and death rates in its Member States using various sources and demographic estimation techniques[2]. The reliability of calculating the completeness of registration in this way clearly depends on the reliability of the independent estimates of crude birth rate (CBR) and crude death rate (CDR).

Completeness of birth registration is calculated as YB = RB/(CBR x P) x 100

YB	Estimated birth registration completeness (%)
RB	Actual number of Registered births
CBR	Crude birth rate, as estimated by the United Nations (per 1000)
P	Total population size (divided by 1000)

Completeness of death registration is calculated as YD = RD/(CDR x P) x 100

YD	Estimated death registration completeness (%)
RD	Actual number of registered deaths
CDR	Crude death rate, as estimated by the United Nations (per1000)
P	Total population size (divided by 1000)

Sample calculation

The United Nations estimates that the CDR for country X in 2005 was 5.4 per 1000 population. The population of country X in 2005 was reported as 69 421 000.

Suppose that, during 2005, the civil registration system registered 280 510 deaths. The completeness of death registration in country X would be estimated as:

YD = 280 510/(5.4 x 69 421) x 100 = 280 510/374, 873 x 100 = 74.8%

---

[1] *Principles and recommendations for a vital statistics system,* Series M, No. 19/Rev. 2. New York, United Nations Statistics Division, 2001. Sales No. 01.XVI.10. Available at: http://unstats.un.org/unsd/publication/SeriesM/SeriesM_19rev2E.pdf

[2] *World population prospects*. New York 2008, United Nations Department of Economic and Social Affairs Statistics Division.

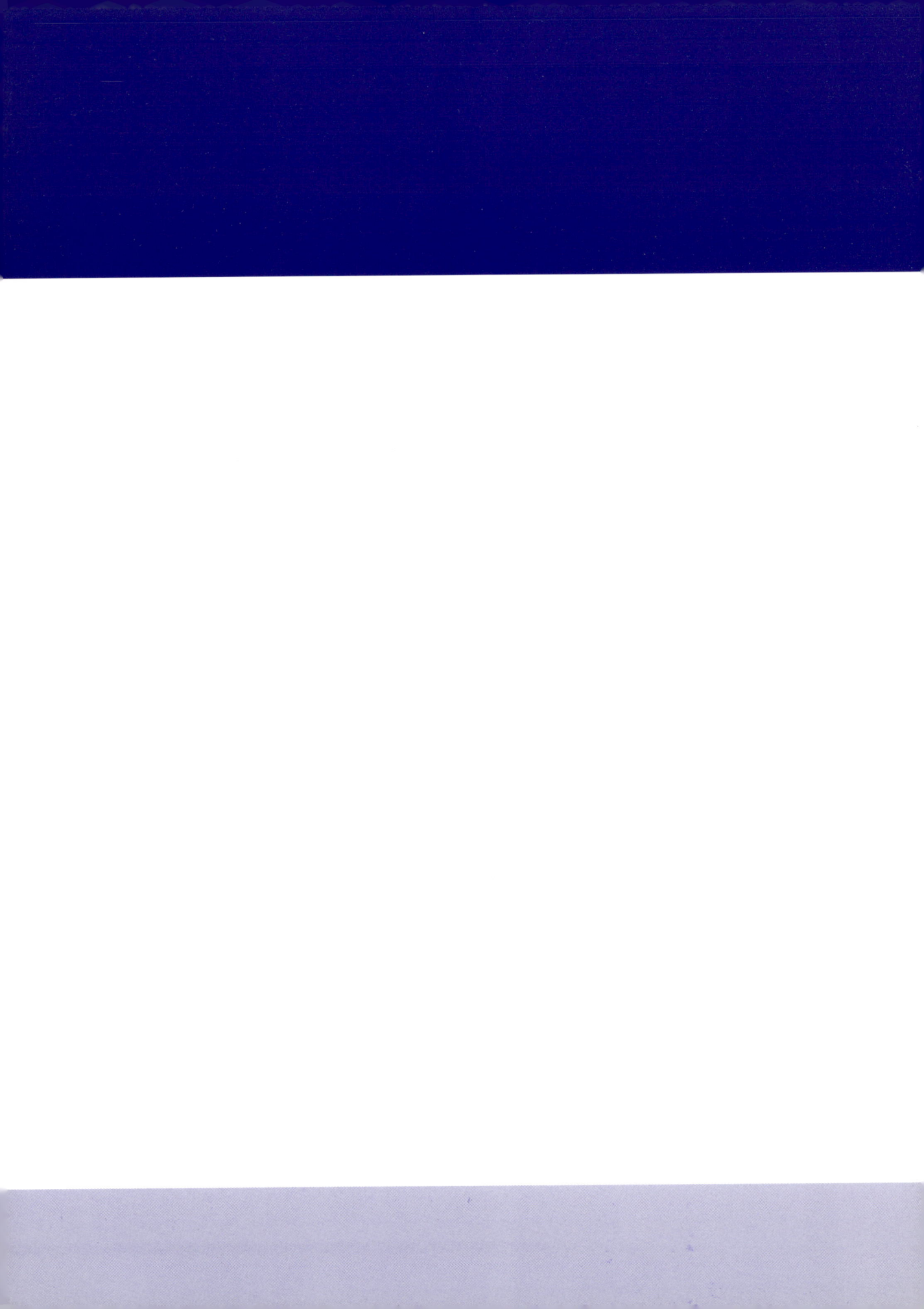